Pharmacology

Medical Examination Review

Pharmacology

Seventh Edition

700 Questions and Answers

Robert A. Woodbury, MD, PhD
Joseph J. Krzanowski, Jr., PhD
Calvin Hanna, PhD
William F. Cantrell, PhD

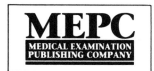

MEPC
MEDICAL EXAMINATION
PUBLISHING COMPANY

Medical Examination Publishing Company
A Division of Elsevier Science Publishing Co., Inc.
655 Avenue of the Americas
New York, NY 10010

Library of Congress Cataloging-in-Publication Data

Medical examination review.
  Includes various editions of some volumes.
  Published 1960–1980 as: Medical examination review book.
  Includes bibliographical references.

  1. Medicine—Examinations, questions, etc.
RC58.M4   610′.76—dc19   61-66847   AACR2   MARC

ISBN 0-444-01586-8

Current printing (last digit):
10 9 8 7 6 5 4 3 2 1

Manufactured in the United States of America

Contents

Preface

This seventh edition of *Medical Examination Review: Pharmacology* has been substantially revised and updated to include current expanding knowledge in pharmacology. It is designed to assist you in preparing for course examinations, National Boards, FLEX, and FMGEMS.

This book contains questions from each important area of pharmacology. The questions are organized in broad categories to give you a representative sampling of the material covered in course work, while helping you to determine those general areas in which you require intensive review.

Explanatory answers, referenced to widely available text and reference books, are included for each question and follow each section. For each question, specific page references to more than one textbook are usually provided, as students may have one textbook and not another. The authors suggest that the student consult the Explanatory Answers immediately after answering several questions so as to discard the incorrect portions of each question and retain the correct knowledge. This book should serve to test your memory and ability to read questions carefully. Do not compromise by simply noting the correct answer and reading the explanatory comments; use the questions to test for areas of weakness. Do not be discouraged if you fail to achieve a high test score, since one benefit from the book is determining where additional review is most needed.

The purpose of this book is to provide a general review of pharmacology. The authors wish to encourage you to consult your textbooks for more in-depth coverage of the subject matter.

Contributors

Robert A. Woodbury, MD, PhD, Professor Emeritus of Pharmacology, Graduate School of Medical Sciences, Medical–Dentistry–Pharmacy–Nursing–Community and Allied Health Professions, University of Tennessee, Memphis, Tennessee

Joseph J. Krzanowski, Jr., PhD, Professor and Acting Chairman of Pharmacology and Therapeutics, University of South Florida College of Medicine, Tampa, Florida

Calvin Hanna, PhD, Professor Emeritus of Pharmacology and Ophthalmology, University of Arkansas College of Medicine, Little Rock, Arkansas

William F. Cantrell, PhD, Professor Emeritus of Pharmacology, Graduate School of Medical Sciences, Medical–Dentistry–Pharmacy–Nursing–Community and Allied Health Professions, University of Tennessee, Memphis, Tennessee

1 Principles of Pharmacology

DIRECTIONS (Questions 1–15): Each of the questions or incomplete statements below is followed by five suggested answers or completions. Select the **one** that is best in each case.

1. Referring to Figure 1, which of the following statements is true?
   A. When curve 1 is in the absence of an antagonist and curve 2 is in the presence of an antagonist, the antagonist is noncompetitive in type
   B. When curve 1 represents the therapeutic effect and curve 2 the lethal effect, the margin of safety is good
   C. When curve 1 represents the therapeutic effect and curve 2 the lethal effect, the therapeutic index is less than 3
   D. When curve 1 represents the therapeutic effect and curve 2 the lethal effect, the therapeutic index is above 10
   E. None of the above

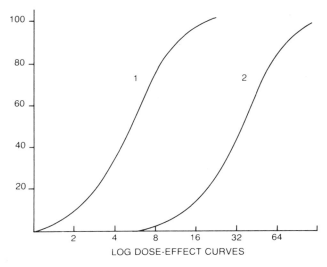

LOG DOSE-EFFECT CURVES

Figure 1

2. All of the following statements are true EXCEPT
   A. the 1906 Pure Food and Drug Act stopped the misla-
      beling and adulteration of drugs
   B. the birth defect, phocomelia, caused by thalidamide
      resulted in the passage in 1962 of the Kefauver-Harris
      Amendment to the Food, Drug, and Cosmetic Act
      requiring proof of safety by research on animals before
      a new drug may be tested in humans
   C. where there is no satisfactory treatment for a life-
      threatening disease, the Food and Drug Administra-
      tion (FDA) may approve limited therapeutic use in
      humans of a new drug showing some efficacy and not
      unreasonable toxicity before data are presented for ap-
      proval of general marketing of the new drug
   D. the 1984 Drug Price Competition and Patent Restric-
      tion Act allowed Abbreviated Drug Application (ADA)
      use for patented drugs to be sold under their generic
      name
   E. once a new drug application (NDA) is approved other
      companies may apply to FDA to market this drug
      under the generic name

3. Which of the following statements is true?
   A. The rate of absorption and the rate of elimination of a drug are usually equal
   B. Plotted on an arithmetic scale, drug elimination follows a straight line
   C. A constant fraction of the drug in the body is eliminated per unit of time
   D. The elimination half-time of a drug is one half of the time required for the elimination of all of the drug
   E. None of the above

4. A drug dose repeated at the elimination half-life, just prior to the third administration, approaches the steady state of further administrations by what percentage?
   A. 50%
   B. 62.5%
   C. 75%
   D. 82.5%
   E. 90%

5. Different lots of a drug preparation have the same bioavailability when they
   A. Are chemically equivalent
   B. Fulfill the same chemical standards as set by regulatory agencies
   C. Yield similar concentrations of the drug in blood and tissues
   D. Have been approved by the Food and Drug Administration (FDA)
   E. Meet the standards set forth by the United States Pharmacopoeia (USP)

6. Passage of drugs through cell membranes is influenced by all of these factors EXCEPT
   A. its pH
   B. its type of action
   C. the amount of protein binding
   D. its lipid solubility
   E. the presence of pores in the membrane

7. Barriers to penetration of drugs into tissues vary in their effectiveness. Which of the following is the most effective barrier?
   A. Placenta early in pregnancy
   B. Placenta late in pregnancy
   C. Brain
   D. Tunica propria of testes
   E. Sertoli cells of testes

8. Passage of drugs across the cell membrane can be through solution in the membrane lipids and is governed by the permeability coefficient times the diffusion area times the concentration gradient. All the following statements are true concerning the passage of drugs EXCEPT
   A. for lipid-soluble (nonpolar) drugs the permeability coefficient is large
   B. for water-soluble (polar) drugs the permeability coefficient is small
   C. the rate of diffusion is independent of the surface area for transfer
   D. the passage of drugs is facilitated by a high concentration gradient
   E. the passage of drugs is facilitated across the lung because of its very large surface area

9. Which of the following statements is true?
   A. The protein-bound drug in the body is the portion of drug that is therapeutically active
   B. Drugs cross the placenta mainly by active transport
   C. The LD_{50} is 50% of the minimum dose that is lethal to animals of a specified species and strain
   D. The LD_{50} is 50% of the average dose that is lethal to animals of a specific species or strain
   E. The maximal intensity of a specified therapeutic effect that a drug is able to produce is referred to as its efficacy

10. Drug permeation, that is, movement of molecules from the site of administration into the body and bodily components, are modified by all of the following mechanisms EXCEPT
    A. lipid diffusion
    B. aqueous diffusion
    C. facilitative diffusion (special carriers)
    D. Henderson-Hasselbalch equation
    E. receptor-mediated endocytosis (Pinocytosis)

11. The signature of a prescription consists of
    A. the names and the amounts of each ingredient
    B. your signature and address
    C. your signature
    D. instructions for the patient as to how and when the medication is to be taken
    E. the quantity to be dispensed

12. Orphan drugs meet all of the following criteria EXCEPT
    A. for patients with rare genetic deficiencies
    B. for the treatment of rare diseases
    C. where the disease population is very young
    D. where the incidence of the disease is too large
    E. where proof of the drug safety must be established in small populations

13. A *new drug application* (NDA) to the FDA requires preclinical safety and toxicity testing including which of the following:
    A. the drug must be shown to be nontoxic in animals
    B. acute toxicity of single doses in at least two species and two routes of administration
    C. mechanism and outline of toxic effects
    D. carcinogenic potential
    E. chronic toxicity for multiple doses in animals for 1 to 2 years

14. The one main goal of phase 1 studies of a new drug application is to determine
    A. the possibility of development of toxic effects
    B. the biologic and therapeutic effects that may be useful in treatment dose range
    C. the required therapeutic dose range
    D. the dosage level where toxic effects may be expected
    E. none of the above

15. All of the following drugs on repeated use may lead to enzyme induction of cytochrome p-450 EXCEPT
    A. isoniazid
    B. ethanol (chronic use)
    C. phenobarbital
    D. phenytoin
    E. digoxin

DIRECTIONS (Questions 16–23): The group of questions below consists of five lettered headings followed by a list of numbered words, phrases, or statements. For each numbered word, phrase, or statement, select the **one** lettered heading that is most closely associated with it. Each lettered heading may be selected once, more than once, or not at all.

Questions 16–18: Drug action is reduced mainly by

    A. oxidation
    B. reduction
    C. hydrolysis
    D. conjugation
    E. excretion unchanged by the kidneys

16. Morphine

17. Phenobarbital

18. Digoxin

Questions 19 – 23: The levels of enzymes involved in drug metabolism is under genetic influence. Match the defect-drug with the clinical consequences

    A. *N*-acetylation defect: isoniazid
    B. Ester hydrolysis defect: tolbutamide
    C. Hydroxylation defect: warfarin
    D. Oxidation defect: debrisoquin (antihypertensive)

19. Cardiotoxicity

20. Bleeding

21. Peripheral neuropathy

22. Prolonged apnea

23. Orthostatic hypotension

DIRECTIONS (Questions 24 and 25): The set of lettered headings below is followed by a list of numbered words or phrases. For each numbered word or phrase select

    A if the item is associated with **A** only
    B if the item is associated with **B** only
    C if the item is associated with both **A** and **B**
    D if the item is associated with neither **A** nor **B**

    A. Physiologic antagonist
    B. Competitive antagonist
    C. Both
    D. Neither

24. Atropine and acetylcholine on heart rate

25. Isoproterenol and acetylcholine on heart rate

DIRECTIONS (Questions 26–37): For each of the questions or incomplete statements below, **one** or **more** of the answers or completions given is correct. Select

    A if only 1, 2, and 3 are correct
    B if only 1 and 3 are correct
    C if only 2 and 4 are correct
    D if only 4 is correct
    E if all are correct

26. Concerning potency and efficacy
    1. potency refers to the maximal effect a drug is capable of producing
    2. efficacy refers to lack of toxicity of a drug
    3. efficacy refers to amount of drug required to produce one half of the maximal effect
    4. their efficacy is more important than their potency when comparing the usefulness of morphine and codeine as analgesics

27. Conditions responsible for excessive or unusual drug effects include
    1. unusual sensitivity, either allergic in nature or an idiosyncratic reaction
    2. administration of the drug too frequently or for a prolonged period of time
    3. the presence of other drugs
    4. the age of the individual

28. The rate of urinary excretion of acidic drugs such as aspirin and barbiturates is increased by
    1. administration of sodium bicarbonate
    2. administration of ammonium chloride
    3. administration of sodium citrate
    4. keeping the urine at neutral pH

29. Drug allergies
1. can develop only when the patient has previously received the drug
2. are more likely to develop in a very young infant
3. are more likely to develop in brunettes
4. can develop when the patient may or may not have been exposed to the drug previously

30. Ionized and/or lipid-insoluble drugs
1. may pass through the small aqueous channels, or pores, of cells of many tissues
2. generally do not gain entry to brain cells
3. cross biologic lipid membranes less readily than do nonionized drugs
4. include such drugs as digitoxin

31. Good correlation exists between lipid solubility and
1. absorption
2. distribution in tissues
3. rate of protein binding
4. duration of action

32. Which of the following statements is (are) true?
1. Teratogenic effects are most likely to develop during the predifferentiation stage of pregnancy (day 1 to day 4)
2. Tachyphylaxis is considered to be present whenever the adult heart rate exceeds the accepted normal range
3. Early in pregnancy the placental membrane is 25 μm in thickness and at term only 2 μm in thickness; this reduces and in some instances eliminates the barrier to nonpenetrating drug molecules
4. The Delaney Amendment of 1958 requires the FDA to restrict from interstate commerce any food additive shown to cause cancer in any animal species at any dose

		Directions Summarized		
A	**B**	**C**	**D**	**E**
1,2,3	1,3	2,4	4	All are
only	only	only	only	correct

33. Drug responsiveness may vary in a single individual to the same drug during treatment course or vary among individuals to the same drug. This change could include
    1. presence of other drugs
    2. very young or very old patients
    3. tolerance to the drug effect
    4. idiosyncratic response to the drug

34. Excretion of drugs via the kidney involves which of the following mechanisms?
    1. Passive glomerulus filtration
    2. Active tubular excretion
    3. Passive tubular reabsorption
    4. Active tubular secretion followed by glomerulus reabsorption

35. Clinical trials evaluating new drugs require
    1. informed consent (where possible)
    2. adverse reactions to the new drug to be immediately reported to the FDA
    3. use of a placebo (where possible) and a standard control drug
    4. the approval of a medical college

36. Drugs may cross cell membranes by
    1. passage through aqueous channels in the membrane
    2. being dissolved in the membrane
    3. active transport, which requires energy
    4. facilitated diffusion, which requires energy

37. The blood–brain barrier
    1. is poorly penetrated by water-soluble drugs
    2. consists of glial cells surrounding the capillaries
    3. is penetrated easily by ether
    4. is penetrated less readily in patients with meningitis

Explanatory Answers

1. E. Noncompetitive (irreversible) antagonists reduce the height of the curve and shift it to the right. The therapeutic index is $LD_{50}/ED_{50} = 32/5.8 = 5.5$ and the margin of safety is $LD_1/ED_{99} = 5.6/16 = 0.35$, which represents a very poor margin of safety. (**Ref.** 1, pp. 13–16, 55–56; **Ref.** 3, p. 12; **Ref.** 6, pp. 45–47; **Ref.** 8, pp. 44–48; **Ref.** 9, pp. 19–29)

2. E. The 1906 Pure Food and Drug Act has been modified to add new goals and to solve new problems. The many amendments were added to protect the public. Because of the great expense involved in developing a new drug which meets the FDA rules and regulations, the new drug is the property of the company that developed it. However, to make some drugs less expensive, the 1984 Drug Price Competition and Patent Application Restriction Action was passed. This Act allows certain older drugs to be marketed by other companies under restrictive conditions. (**Ref.** 1, pp. 51–58; **Ref.** 8, pp. 74–75)

3. C. Drug elimination follows an exponential decay curve when plotted on an arithmetic scale. Elimination half-life is the time required for one half of the drug to be eliminated. It takes several elimination half-times for the body to rid itself of all of the drug. (**Ref.** 3, pp. 17–18; **Ref.** 6, pp. 26–27; **Ref.** 8, pp. 23–25; **Ref.** 9, pp. 57–65)

4. C. With two doses, 75% of the plateau blood level will be reached. With antibiotics and a few other drugs, the first dose is frequently doubled so that the plateau (steady state) is approached with the first dose. (**Ref.** 3, pp. 17–18; **Ref.** 6, pp. 26–29; **Ref.** 8, pp. 23–25; **Ref.** 9, pp. 17–20)

5. C. Several preparations may be composed of the same chemicals and meet regulatory chemical standards but differ in particle size or crystalline form so that rate and amount of absorption differ. Consequently, they would not possess the same bioavailability. (**Ref.** 3, p. 23)

6. B. All of the factors listed, except the type of action of a drug, influence the passage of drugs through cell membranes; however, highly lipid-soluble drugs can enter the central nervous system (CNS) even though pores are not present. Aqueous-soluble drugs encounter a barrier in the absence of pores. (**Ref.** 1, p. 15; **Ref.** 2, pp. 25–27; **Ref.** 6, pp. 3–6; **Ref.** 8, pp. 3–5; **Ref.** 9, pp. 22–26)

7. E. Sertoli cells of the testes are tightly packed together, forming an effective barrier to drug penetration. (**Ref.** 2, p. 32)

8. C. In Fick's law of diffusion: flux = permeability coefficient × diffusion area × concentration gradient. The coefficient for a nonpolar drug is large and for polar drugs is small. A high concentration gradient and a large surface area would facilitate the passage of drugs across a membrane or tissue. (**Ref.** 1, pp. 2–3; **Ref.** 9, pp. 24–26, 30)

9. E. Only an unbound drug is therapeutically active. Drugs readily diffuse across the placenta. The LD_{50} is that dose which is lethal to 50% of the animals. Efficacy refers to the potential maximal therapeutic effect. (**Ref.** 1, pp. 23–25; **Ref.** 6, p. 12; **Ref.** 9, pp. 22, 34)

10. D. The Henderson-Hasselbalch equation has to do with the ionization of weak acids and bases. The degree of ionization is one factor that influences the water solubility of a drug. The diffusion, or movement process, is dependent on a number of factors including lipid, water, facilitative diffusions, and pinocytosis. (**Ref.** 1, pp. 2–4; **Ref.** 8, p. 4; **Ref.** 9, pp. 21–23)

11. D. In a prescription, the signature is the instructions for the patient; the name and amount of each ingredient is known as the inscription; the quantity to be dispensed is known as the subscription. (**Ref.** 6, pp. 1653–1654; **Ref.** 8, p. 1640; **Ref.** 9, p. 108)

12. D. Under normal FDA-NDA rules drugs designed to benefit a small segment of a population would be far more expensive to market than the income generated by the sales to such a small market. The Orphan Drug Act was designed to help industry develop these drugs for the limited market. (**Ref.** 1, p. 57; **Ref.** 8, pp. 74–78)

13. A. Toxicity of a new drug must be tested in animals to reveal possible toxicities to be expected in humans after an overdose. There are exceptions to this rule, such as when a new drug is to be applied to restricted areas in very small amounts; however, even under these conditions toxicity testing in animals is necessary to define the possible toxicity should the drug be accidentally ingested or used in another manner. (**Ref.** 1, pp. 53–55; **Ref.** 8, pp. 54–55)

14. B. The evaluation of drugs in phase I should provide information in as many areas as can be reasonably expected so that dose range and possible toxic effects may be investigated, but the main goal is to determine whether the drug is potentially useful in therapy. (**Ref.** 1, pp. 56–57; **Ref.** 6, pp. 58–59; **Ref.** 8, pp. 74–78; **Ref.** 9, pp. 111–112)

15. E. Induced cytochrome P-450 activity may increase the metabolism of the drug that stimulated the enzyme activity. Isoniazid, chronic ethanol use, phenobarbital, and phenytoin are some of the main drugs that induce cytochrome P-450 activity. (**Ref.** 1, pp. 43–45; **Ref.** 2, pp. 43–47; **Ref.** 6, pp. 58–59; **Ref.** 8, pp. 74–78; **Ref.** 9, pp. 111–112)

16. D. In humans, morphine is eliminated mainly by conjugation. (**Ref.** 1, pp. 44; **Ref.** 6, pp. 14, 20–21; **Ref.** 8, pp. 14–15)

17. A. Oxidation of phenobarbi.̃al into hydroxyphenobarbital accounts for most of the cessation of its action, though as much as 25% may be excreted by the kidneys. (**Ref.** 1, p. 44; **Ref.** 6, pp. 14, 455; **Ref.** 8, pp. 14–15; **Ref.** 9, p. 42)

18. E. Approximately two thirds of digoxin is excreted unchanged by the kidneys. This accounts for its shorter duration of action as compared with digitoxin, which is mainly metabolized by the liver. (**Ref.** 1, p. 44; **Ref.** 2, pp. 276–277; **Ref.** 3, pp. 82, 428, 765; **Ref.** 6, pp. 734–735; **Ref.** 8, pp. 827–828)

19. B. The tolbutamide package insert contains a warning about cardiotoxicity. The University Group Diabetes Program report suggested that tolbutamide has a toxic effect on the heart since some of the patients had heart attacks during their study. This might occur when a patient is given a large dose of tolbutamide. In patients with a genetic defect of ester hydrolysis the tolbutamide would persist longer and a cumulative effect could occur resulting in hypoglycemia and possibly cardiotoxicity. (**Ref.** 1, pp. 525–526; **Ref.** 8, p. 1486)

20. C. Warfarin is an anticoagulant and a genetic defect in its inactivation would require the use of smaller than average doses of the drug. (**Ref.** 1, pp. 47–48; **Ref.** 2, p. 59; **Ref.** 8, p. 73)

21. A. Increased blood levels of isoniazid would lead to a variety of toxic effects on the nervous system including insomnia, muscle twitching, and peripheral neuritis. (**Ref.** 1, p. 47; **Ref.** 2, p. 709)

22. E. Succinylcholine was one of the first drugs discovered where a genetic defect in metabolism greatly altered the drug's use. A defect in pseudocholinesterase resulted in prolonging the action of succinylcholine from minutes to hours. (**Ref.** 1, pp. 47–48; **Ref.** 2, p. 239; **Ref.** 8, p. 73)

23. D. Debrisoquin is an antihypertensive-vasodilator drug. When the blood levels of the drug are increased due to a genetic defect in oxidation the side effect is orthostatic hypotension. (**Ref.** 1, pp. 47–48)

24. B. Atropine, by its competitive action against acetylcholine on cholinergic receptors, depending on the dose given, can reduce or prevent the bradycardia otherwise produced by acetylcholine. Some other competitive antagonists are propranolol with β-adrenergic agonists and naloxone with opiates. (**Ref.** 1, p. 74; **Ref.** 2, pp. 18, 195; **Ref.** 3, pp. 12, 116, 183; **Ref.** 6, pp. 132–134, 160)

25. A. Isoproterenol causes tachycardia, and acetylcholine causes bradycardia. They are antagonistic to each other, but at different sites. (**Ref.** 3, p. 47; **Ref.** 6, pp. 132–134, 160)

26. D. Confusion sometimes occurs between potency and efficacy. Potency is determined by finding the dose required to produce a given effect. Comparison of drug potency is relatively unimportant unless the ratio for doses is different for potency and toxic effects. Comparison of drugs for efficacy is important because efficacy refers to the maximal therapeutic effect which can be obtained. In severe pain, codeine is ineffective, even with increased doses. **(Ref.** 1, p. 56; **Ref.** 3, p. 11; **Ref.** 6, pp. 44–45; **Ref.** 8, p. 67; **Ref.** 9, pp. 14–16)

27. E. These are only a few of the conditions that modify drug effects. Administration of a drug for a prolonged period can cause increased effects due to accumulation of the drug or due to cumulative effects without any increased drug levels, or it may cause decreased actions due to tolerance. Infants and elderly patients are more sensitive to many drugs, particularly those that depress the central nervous system. **(Ref.** 1, pp. 47–53; **Ref.** 3, pp. 28, 36, 50, 57, 68, 70, 75; **Ref.** 6, pp. 52, 1595; **Ref.** 8, p. 17; **Ref.** 9, pp. 59–63)

28. B. Sodium bicarbonate and sodium citrate cause the urine to become alkaline, thereby reducing reabsorption of acidic drugs by the tubules. Excretion, therefore, is increased. **(Ref.** 2, p. 556; **Ref.** 3, pp. 23–24, 739; **Ref.** 8, p. 4; **Ref.** 9, pp. 59–63)

29. D. Usually the drug has been administered previously; however, cross-sensitivity is not uncommon; i.e., a patient allergic to procaine after previously receiving procaine is also allergic to other ester-linkage local anesthetics such as piperocaine. **(Ref.** 1, p. 727; **Ref.** 2, p. 459; **Ref.** 3, pp. 44, 373; **Ref.** 6, pp. 1595–1596)

30. A. Ionized and/or lipid-insoluble drugs do reach most cells by passage through pores; however, this is not the case for brain cells because of the blood–brain barrier. **(Ref.** 1, pp. 1–6; **Ref.** 2, pp. 23–26, 34–35; **Ref.** 3, pp. 14, 22; **Ref.** 6, p. 11; **Ref.** 8, p. 4; **Ref.** 9, pp. 21–24)

31. E. Regarding lipid-soluble drugs, the greater the lipid solubility, the more rapidly it is absorbed, the more rapidly it enters the

CNS, the more rapidly it is bound to proteins, and the shorter is the duration of action. (**Ref.** 1, p. 2; **Ref.** 3, pp. 21–23; **Ref.** 6, pp. 4, 11; **Ref.** 9, pp. 20–24)

32. D. The embryonic period (day 15 to day 56) is the period where the danger of teratogenic effects is greatest. Tachyphylaxis is rapidly developing tolerance. The placental barrier to nonpenetrating drugs remains present throughout pregnancy. The cyclamates were the "victim" of the Delaney Amendment, even though very large doses were given to the test animals. (**Ref.** 2, pp. 35, 90, 93–94; **Ref.** 8, p. 13; **Ref.** 9, pp. 37–38)

33. E. The variation of drug response during a single course of therapy and variations among individuals are due to many factors including drug interactions, age, sex, pregnancy, weight, and unexpected sensitivity and responses. (**Ref.** 1, p. 25; **Ref.** 9, pp. 79–81)

34. A. When a drug is excreted by the kidneys, one or more of the following are responsible: glomerular filtration, active tubular secretion, and passive tubular reabsorption. (**Ref.** 1, p. 6; **Ref.** 2, pp. 271–277; **Ref.** 8, p. 18; **Ref.** 9, pp. 59–63)

35. A. Many clinical trials of new drugs are conducted by medical college faculty, although the FDA does not require the input of medical college faculties. However, it does require informed patient consent, reports of adverse effects, and, where possible, the use of a placebo and a standard control drug for comparison to make the study more valid. (**Ref.** 1, pp. 54–58; **Ref.** 2, pp. 127–132; **Ref.** 8, pp. 74–78; **Ref.** 9, pp. 50–52, 55–56, 110)

36. A. Facilitated diffusion does occur but it does not require expenditure of energy. However, it does show selectivity and the mechanism is capable of saturation. (**Ref.** 1, pp. 2–4; **Ref.** 3, pp. 14–15; **Ref.** 8, pp. 4–5)

37. A. Penicillin does not penetrate the blood–brain barrier under normal conditions; however, the inflammation present in meningitis modifies its permeability, permitting the penetration by penicillin. (**Ref.** 1, pp. 555–556; **Ref.** 3, p. 22; **Ref.** 6, p. 1122; **Ref.** 8, p. 11; **Ref.** 9, p. 26)

2 Water, Electrolytes, and Diuretics

DIRECTIONS (Questions 38–40): Each of the questions or incomplete statements below is followed by five suggested answers or completions. Select the **one** that is best in each case.

38. All of the following statements about furosemide are correct EXCEPT
    A. toxic effects are unusual, but include gastrointestinal distress, skin rash, thrombocytopenia, neutropenia, and hypochloremia
    B. its primary effect is inhibition of chloride reabsorption in the ascending limb of the loop of Henle
    C. it may produce hypovolemia shock due to an exaggerated response
    D. it is one of the most potent diuretic drugs
    E. when given in high doses it may produce metabolic acidosis because it inhibits H^+ secretion in the distal tubule

39. Undesirable side effects of thiazide diuretics include all of the following EXCEPT
    A. with prolonged use, azotemia may occur
    B. hyperglycemia
    C. reduced renal blood flow and glomerular filtration rate
    D. potassium retention with excess water loss
    E. cholestatic hepatitis

40. All of the following statements about mannitol are correct EXCEPT
   A. it produces diuresis in the presence of reduced glomerular filtration rate
   B. it is filterable and poorly reabsorbed in the renal tubules
   C. it produces very little, if any, change in the acid–base balance
   D. it is used to measure the rate of glomerulus filtration
   E. it is the choice diuretic to treat chronic pulmonary edema

---

DIRECTIONS (Questions 41 and 42): The group of questions below consists of five lettered headings followed by a list of numbered words or phrases. For each numbered word or phrase, select the **one** lettered heading that is most closely associated with it. Each lettered heading may be selected once, more than once, or not at all.

   A. Glomerulus
   B. Proximal tubule
   C. Loop of Henle
   D. Distal tubule
   E. Collecting tubule

41. Triamterene

42. Vasopressin on the V_2 receptors of the kidney

DIRECTIONS (Questions 43–47): Each set of lettered headings below is followed by a list of numbered words or phrases. For each numbered word or phrase select

A   if the item is associated with **A** only
B   if the item is associated with **B** only
C   if the item is associated with both **A** and **B**
D   if the item is associated with neither **A** nor **B**

Questions 43 and 44:

A. Increased response to a diuretic agent
B. Improved circulation of blood
C. Both
D. Neither

43. Bed rest and low-salt diet in an edematous individual

44. Frequent blood transfusions in a patient with hypoproteinemia

Questions 45–47:

A. Used to reduce intraocular pressure
B. Preferred diuretic in patients with edema due to cirrhosis of the liver
C. Both
D. Neither

45. Acetazolamide

46. Furosemide

47. Spironolactone

DIRECTIONS (Questions 48–50): For each of the questions or incomplete statements below, **one** or **more** of the answers or completions given is correct. Select

A if only 1, 2, and 3 are correct
B if only 1 and 3 are correct
C if only 2 and 4 are correct
D if only 4 is correct
E if all are correct

48. The most common toxic effect(s) of
1. furosemide are those resulting from abnormal electrolyte levels
2. triamterene are those associated with carbonic anhydrase inhibition
3. mannitol is acute increase of extracellular fluid
4. thiazides are those associated with hyperkalemia

49. Concerning diuretics
1. in patients with renal failure ethacrynic acid given intravenously with aminoglycosides has caused permanent hearing loss
2. furosemide can decrease water reabsorption whereas thiazides do not depress water reabsorption
3. amiloride and triamterene are antikaliuretic diuretics
4. in the treatment of hypertension without renal failure, thiazides are preferred over loop diuretics

50. Concerning water, electrolytes, and diuretics
1. spironolactone acts as an aldosterone antagonist
2. the most frequent side effects of spironolactone are due to hyperkalemia
3. in metabolic acidosis the kidneys are important organs in bringing about a normal acid–base balance
4. potential side effects of triamterene include nausea, dizziness, and leg cramps

Explanatory Answers

38. E. Furosemide and ethacrynic acid, known as high-ceiling or loop diuretics, can produce metabolic alkalosis, not acidosis; they are excreted mainly in the urine by the proximal tubules and inhibit sodium and chloride reabsorption in the ascending loop of Henle. (**Ref.** 3, p. 489; **Ref.** 4, p. 484; **Ref.** 6, pp. 896–898; **Ref.** 8, pp. 721–723)

39. D. Hypokalemia, not hyperkalemia, is the most common adverse effect of the thiazides. To keep the potassium levels normal, therapy should include one or more of the following: (1) diet rich in fruits and vegetables, (2) potassium chloride taken orally daily, or (3) combination with potassium-sparing diuretics. (**Ref.** 3, pp. 485–486; **Ref.** 4, p. 2524; **Ref.** 6, pp. 873–874, 892–895)

40. E. Because mannitol must be given intravenously, its use as a diuretic is very limited. Administered as a hypertonic solution, it reduces elevated intracranial pressure without a rebound increase in pressure; it also increases the extracellular volume so its use is contraindicated in patients with cardiac decompensation. (**Ref.** 3, pp. 482–483; **Ref.** 6, pp. 888–889; **Ref.** 8, p. 714)

41. D. Triamterene, by its action on the distal tubules, inhibits sodium reabsorption and potassium secretion. Therefore, in combination with the thiazides, triamterene prevents the hypokalemic effects of the thiazides. (**Ref.** 3, pp. 481, 491; **Ref.** 8, p. 727)

42. E. Vasopressin acting on the V_2 receptors in the collecting tubules causes them to become permeable to water. Because the urine at this site is hypotonic, water is reabsorbed by osmosis. (**Ref.** 8, pp. 736, 737)

43. C. Bed rest reduces the demand on the heart, improving circulation and facilitating reabsorption of edematous fluid, permitting greater response to diuretics. (**Ref.** 3, pp. 478–479)

44. A. Circulation and renal flow may be adequate in patients with hypoproteinemia; however, transfusions will restore proper plasma protein levels permitting osmotic forces to return extravascular fluid to the vascular space, thereby increasing diuresis by the diuretics. (**Ref. 3**, pp. 478, 480)

45. A. Acetazolamide is occasionally used as a diuretic. Its principle use is to reduce intraocular pressure in simple glaucoma. Administered orally, 250 mg, one to four times daily, it decreases formation of aqueous humor by inhibiting carbonic anhydrase in the ciliary process. (**Ref. 8**, pp. 736, 737)

46. D. Although furosemide is a potent diuretic, aldosterone inhibitors are the preferred diuretics in patients with cirrhosis of the liver. High-ceiling diuretics, however, are the drugs of choice for acute pulmonary edema. (**Ref. 3**, pp. 489, 490; **Ref. 8**, p. 725)

47. B. In cirrhosis of the liver, where sodium reabsorption and potassium excretion are high due to elevated aldosterone levels, spironolactone, an aldosterone antagonist, reduces the edema very effectively. (**Ref. 3**, p. 490; **Ref. 8**, pp. 725, 727)

48. B. Triamterene does not inhibit carbonic anhydrase. Prolonged administration of furosemide may also produce serious hypovolemia. (**Ref. 8**, pp. 715, 721, 724, 727, 730)

49. E. Furosemide may also cause reduced formation of various blood cells, gastrointestinal problems, skin rashes, paresis, and hepatic dysfunctions. Thiazides are used extensively in antihypertensive therapy acting directly and also indirectly by increasing the action of other antihypertensive drugs. Thiazides should be used cautiously in patients with diabetes mellitus as they can decrease insulin secretion, increase glycogenolysis, and decrease glycogenesis. (**Ref. 8**, pp. 721, 727, 731, 785–788)

50. E. In metabolic acidosis the kidneys completely reabsorb sodium bicarbonate and excrete fixed anions combined with NH rather than Na. (**Ref. 8**, pp. 711, 725–726, 728)

3 Drugs Affecting the Autonomic Nervous System

DIRECTIONS (Questions 51–93): Each of the questions or incomplete statements below is followed by five suggested answers or completions. Select the **one** that is best in each case.

51. The mechanism of action of prazosin involves
    A. activation of β_1-receptors only
    B. a specific activation of α_2-receptors
    C. a blockade of α_1-receptors
    D. an elimination of β_2 effects
    E. production of a nonequilibrium α-adrenergic blockade

52. The distinguishing feature of nadolol among the β-adrenergic blocking agents is
    A. cardioselectivity
    B. blockade of β_2-receptors only
    C. duration of action
    D. development of a nonequilibrium blockade
    E. effectiveness in therapeutic management of bronchial asthma

53. Noncatecholamine adrenergic amines differ from catecholamines in that they
    A. have a short duration of action
    B. are not effective if administered orally
    C. do not act indirectly, but usually combine directly with adrenergic receptors of the α_1 and β_2 subtypes
    D. tend to have greater central nervous system (CNS) effects following oral administration
    E. are metabolized at a more rapid rate

54. Adrenergic amines might be employed therapeutically for all of the following conditions EXCEPT
    A. relief of symptoms of acute hypersensitivity reactions to drugs
    B. production of miosis and cycloplegia
    C. narcolepsy
    D. activation of the vagal reflex mechanism in paroxysmal atrial tachycardia
    E. reduction of nasal congestion for temporary relief from upper respiratory infections

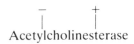

55. Above is a diagrammatic representation of sites of drug interaction on the acetylcholinesterase enzyme. All of the following statements are true EXCEPT
    A. acetylcholine is hydrolyzed after combination with the esteratic (+) and anionic (−) sites
    B. neostigmine carbamylates the esteratic (+) site and is slowly hydrolyzed
    C. irreversible inhibitors of the enzyme act by forming an alkylphosphorylation of the anionic site (−)
    D. regeneration of the enzyme occurs when oximes attach to the anionic site (−) and exert a nucleophilic attack on the phosphorus
    E. the binding of diisopropyl fluorophosphate (DFP) to the esteratic site (+) undergoes an "aging" process

56. Postoperative urinary retention may be best treated with
    A. DFP
    B. carbachol
    C. ephedrine
    D. bethanechol
    E. atropine

57. The enhanced pressor response to norepinephrine in humans after the administration of amitriptyline is most likely caused by
    A. increased sensitivity of tissue to norepinephrine
    B. increased activity of catechol-O-methyltransferase (COMT)
    C. interference with uptake of norepinephrine into adrenergic nerves
    D. increased activity of monoamine oxidase
    E. decreased destruction of norepinephrine by metabolic enzymes

58. The major pathway for the removal of norepinephrine released from nerves into the synaptic gap is
    A. degradation by monoamine oxidase
    B. uptake into adrenergic nerve (uptake$_1$)
    C. diffusion from the synapse into the general circulation
    D. binding with plasma proteins
    E. uptake into smooth muscle cells of spleen, heart, and kidney (uptake$_2$)

59. Which of the following is an accepted therapeutic use of epinephrine?
    A. Combinations with local anesthetics in 1 : 1000 concentrations
    B. Treatment of pheochromocytoma
    C. IV infusion in cases of hemorrhagic shock
    D. Treatment of cardiac asthma
    E. Treatment of acute hypersensitivity reaction to drugs

60. Which of the following is the correct sequence for norepinephrine synthesis in humans?
    A. Tyrosine (hydroxylase) → dopamine (methyltransferase) → dopa (decarboxylase) → norepinephrine
    B. Tyrosine (hydroxylase) → dopa (decarboxylase) → dopamine (methyltransferase) → norepinephrine
    C. Tyrosine (hydroxylase) → dopa (decarboxylase) → dopamine (β-hydroxylase) → epinephrine (methyltransferase) → norepinephrine
    D. Tyrosine (hydroxylase) → dopa (decarboxylase) → dopamine (β-hydroxylase) → norepinephrine
    E. Tyrosine (hydroxylase) → dopamine (decarboxylase) → dopa (methyltransferase) → epinephrine (β-hydroxylase) → norepinephrine

61. Timolol
    A. is an anticholinesterase
    B. is a cholinergic drug
    C. is a β-adrenergic antagonist
    D. is principally an α-adrenergic agonist with minimal β-adrenergic agonist activity
    E. causes mydriasis and ciliary spasm fixed for near vision

62. The mechanism of action of hemicholinium
    A. prevents the liberation of acetylcholine (ACh)
    B. mimics the action of ACh
    C. blocks the transport system responsible for choline accumulation in terminals of cholinergic fibers
    D. inactivates cholinesterase of the ganglia
    E. prevents the interaction between ACh and the receptor sites

63. The mechanism of action of botulinus toxin
    A. mimics ACh
    B. prevents release of ACh
    C. potentiates action of cholinesterase
    D. inhibits action of cholinesterase
    E. prevents the synthesis of ACh

64. Which of the following statements is true regarding sympathomimetic amines?

    A. Phenylephrine or methoxamine may successfully end attacks of paroxysmal atrial or nodal tachycardia by vagal reflex without causing significant cardiac stimulation

    B. The pressor action of metaraminol is mainly indirect and is dependent upon epinephrine release

    C. Nylidrin and isoxsuprine are typical α-receptor stimulators

    D. The injection of epinephrine will cause a marked decrease in plasma free fatty acids but only in the presence of a functioning adrenal gland

    E. Epinephrine produces an increase in coronary blood flow, which accounts for its usefulness in relieving precordial pain in anginal attacks

65. Which drug causes the following side effects: dry mouth, visual disturbances (mydriasis, photophobia, blurred vision due to cycloplegia), hypotension, marked postural hypotension, decreased or absent potentia, occasional diarrhea interspersed with periods of intestinal paralysis, eructation, and urinary retention?

    A. Neostigmine

    B. Guanethidine

    C. Reserpine

    D. Phenylephrine

    E. Mecamylamine

66. Concerning the metabolism of epinephrine and nor-epinephrine
    A. under normal conditions, the enzymes MAO and COMT are responsible for the termination of the actions of epinephrine and norepinephrine
    B. the enzyme COMT is mainly responsible for the metabolism of epinephrine and norepinephrine into 3,4-dihydroxymandelic acid
    C. one end-metabolic product of epinephrine and norepinephrine is 3-methoxy-4-hydroxymandelic acid (vanillylmandelic acid or VMA)
    D. metanephrine glucuronide is a precursor of VMA
    E. guanethidine causes enzyme induction of MAO and COMT

67. Which of the following autonomic drugs decreases the amount of norepinephrine released by adrenergic nerves per stimulus, but in a single dose does not cause norepinephrine depletion, instead, it may increase tissue norepinephrine content; accumulates in adrenergic nerves; and is a local anesthetic?
    A. α-Methyldopa
    B. Veratrum
    C. Reserpine
    D. Phenoxybenzamine
    E. Bretylium

68. Which of the following statements is true concerning sympathomimetic agents?
  A. On the heart, the action of epinephrine is excitatory via α_1-receptors and inhibitory via β_1-receptors
  B. On intestinal smooth muscle, the action of epinephrine is excitatory via β_2-receptors and inhibitory via α_2-receptors
  C. The adrenal medulla secretes epinephrine in response to injected acetylcholine, and this response is blocked by hexamethonium
  D. The action of MAO and COMT to terminate the action of the sympathetic transmitter is entirely analogous to the action of acetylcholinesterase to terminate the action of acetylcholine on the parasympathetic side
  E. Addiction and tolerance are rarely seen with amphetamine

69. All of the following statements are true regarding treatment of bronchial asthma EXCEPT
  A. epinephrine gives relief mainly by relaxing bronchial smooth muscle, β_2-receptor activation
  B. smaller doses of drug given early in an attack are more effective than larger doses given later
  C. tolerance to epinephrine can be a problem in chronic bronchial asthma
  D. tolerance to epinephrine should be treated with infusion of epinephrine
  E. measures designed to remove inspissated mucus plugs are important

70. Regarding the treatment of Parkinson's disease, all of the following statements are true EXCEPT
  A. the parkinsonian patient has a reduced amount of dopamine in basal ganglia
  B. reserpine depletes dopamine and may produce parkinsonlike symptoms
  C. phenothiazines antagonize catecholamines and cause parkinsonian side effects
  D. dopamine readily crosses the blood–brain barrier
  E. impressive improvement occurs in patients with doses of L-dopa of up to 8 g daily

71. All of the following statements are true concerning the "amine pump," or uptake mechanism, of the adrenergic nerve terminals EXCEPT
    A. it is not highly specific for norepinephrine
    B. it will take up metaraminol in significant amounts
    C. it will take up and accumulate "false transmitters"
    D. it will not take up 6-hydroxydopamine
    E. it is blocked by imipramine

72. Which of the following statements concerning nicotinic and muscarinic receptors is FALSE?
    A. Nicotine has the property of being both a cholinergic receptor stimulant and a blocking agent
    B. The nicotinic receptors of autonomic ganglia and skeletal muscle are not entirely identical
    C. It is now accepted that autonomic ganglion cells have both nicotinic and muscarinic receptors
    D. Atropine blocks the excitatory muscarinic actions of acetylcholine, but not the inhibitory actions
    E. Methacholine may cause a rise of blood pressure in the patient with adrenal medullary tumor

73. All of the following are α-adrenergic blockers EXCEPT
    A. ergotoxine
    B. tolazoline
    C. ergonovine
    D. dibenamine
    E. phentolamine

74. All of the following are typical cholinergic effects EXCEPT
    A. a decrease in heart rate
    B. an increase in atrial–ventrical (A–V) conduction time
    C. an increase in secretion of sweat
    D. an increase in pupillary diameter
    E. a contraction of bronchial muscle

75. Acetylcholine is the neurotransmitter at all of the following sites EXCEPT
    A. muscarinic receptor sites
    B. nicotinic$_1$ receptor sites
    C. nicotinic$_2$ receptor sites
    D. adrenergic ganglia
    E. α_2-adrenergic receptor sites

76. The process referred to as uptake$_2$
    A. is inhibited by cocaine
    B. causes decreased release of norepinephrine
    C. is also called extraneuronal uptake
    D. is blocked by imipramine
    E. blocks the action of tyramine

77. All of the following statements are true regarding nicotine EXCEPT
    A. nicotine is an alkaloid which is readily absorbed through the skin
    B. nicotine both stimulates and blocks receptor sites
    C. the action of nicotine is limited to skeletal muscle paralysis
    D. the effects of toxic doses of nicotine can be predicted by knowing the predominant innervation of an organ
    E. administration of nicotine would be expected to cause release of epinephrine from the adrenal gland

78. Administration of an infusion of norepinephrine to a person will result in
    A. an increase in peripheral resistance
    B. a decrease in A – V transmission
    C. an increase in heart rate
    D. a decrease in mean blood pressure
    E. a decrease in diastolic blood pressure

79. Epinephrine
    A. is a potent stimulant of respiration
    B. inhibits the release of inflammatory mediators from mast cells
    C. causes airway smooth muscle to contract
    D. may cause hypoglycemia
    E. produces miosis

80. Concerning the molecular structure of adrenergic receptors
   A. α_2-adrenergic receptors stimulate adenylyl cyclase
   B. all β-adrenergic receptors inhibit adenylyl cyclase
   C. G_i proteins act to inhibit adenylyl cyclase following activation of α_2-receptors
   D. β_1-adrenergic receptors interact with a G protein called G_i
   E. β_2-adrenergic receptors stimulate G_i

81. Desensitization to catecholamines may be caused by all of the following EXCEPT
   A. phosphorylation of receptors
   B. internalization of receptors
   C. alteration of G proteins
   D. alterations in cyclic nucleotide phosphodiesterase
   E. stimulation or acceleration of cAMP production

82. Human uterine smooth muscle
   A. is relaxed by muscarinic receptor activation
   B. is relaxed by α-adrenergic receptor activation
   C. may be relaxed by β_2-receptor activation
   D. can be inhibited by α-receptor activation at parturition
   E. relaxes when β_2 agonists are given to nonpregnant patients

83. Dopamine
   A. causes renal vasodilation through D_1-receptors
   B. reduces peripheral resistance when administered in high concentrations
   C. has minimal β_1 effects on the heart
   D. inactivates adenylyl cyclase
   E. rapidly enters the CNS

84. β_2-adrenergic agonists
   A. cause significant skeletal muscle relaxation as a side effect
   B. produce reduced levels of glucose in the blood
   C. cause arrhythmias in most patients
   D. may cause the insulin requirement to increase in diabetic patients
   E. usually causes significant and troublesome tolerance in most patients

85. Ipratropium
  A. is a bronchoconstrictor
  B. must be administered orally
  C. should not be given to asthmatic patients
  D. is a quaternary compound
  E. usually causes excessive salivation

86. In the following list all are correct pairings EXCEPT
  A. labetalol/lacks α_2 activity
  B. pindolol/intrinsic sympathomimetic activity
  C. bitolterol/prodrug
  D. tyramine/indirect acting amine
  E. metoprolol/specific β_2 agonist

87. Antimuscarinic agents
  A. are difficult to use without troublesome side effects
  B. effectively decrease gastric acid secretion in low doses
  C. produce mydriasis without cycloplegia
  D. can be given to produce cycloplegia without mydriasis
  E. are relatively nontoxic and large doses can be safely employed

88. Cholinergic excess
  A. may occur as a result of ingestion of the mushroom *Amanita phalloidies*
  B. in the central nervous system (CNS) can be effectively treated with ipratropium
  C. caused by organophosphates can be reversed if pralidoxime is administered immediately after organophosphate ingestion
  D. is almost always produced by ingestion of *Amanita muscaria*
  E. in the CNS is treated with pralidoxime

89. Regarding anticholinesterase activity, all of the following statements are true EXCEPT
    A. neostigmine is a quaternary amine
    B. physostigmine enters into the CNS
    C. both neostigmine and physostigmine inhibit the hydrolysis of acetylcholine
    D. neostigmine can cause direct cholinergic activation of skeletal muscle
    E. neostigmine and physostigmine are considered to be irreversible agents

90. Regarding cholinoceptive sites
    A. actions of acetylcholine are potentiated by scopolamine
    B. bethanechol is potentiated by neostigmine
    C. curare will inhibit the effectiveness of neostigmine at the neuromuscular junction
    D. hexamethonium is a neuromuscular blocker
    E. muscarinic receptors are not considered cholinoceptive

91. All of the following statements are true for pilocarpine EXCEPT
    A. causes contraction of the intestinal tract
    B. may be used to treat asthma
    C. induces vasodilation
    D. is effective for open-angle glaucoma
    E. produces marked diaphoresis (sweating)

92. The effects of acetylcholine or cholinergic agonists on the myocardium include
    A. counteraction of the indirect effect of digitalis
    B. decreased contractile force development
    C. decreased A-V conduction time
    D. stimulation of the sinoatrial (SA) node
    E. increased speed of A-V conduction

93. Ganglionic blockade would most likely produce
    A. increased urinary frequency
    B. decreased heart rate
    C. salivation
    D. mydriasis
    E. vasoconstriction

DIRECTIONS (Questions 94–155): Each group of questions below consists of five lettered headings followed by a list of numbered words, phrases, or statements. For each numbered word, phrase, or statement, select the **one** lettered heading that is most closely associated with it. Each lettered heading may be selected once, more than once, or not at all.

Questions 94–97:

    A. Phentolamine
    B. Prazosin
    C. Phenoxybenzamine
    D. Clonidine
    E. Yohimbine

94. An adrenergic blocking agent which has a long duration of action and which is not specific for α-receptors

95. A specific antagonist of α_2-adrenergic receptors

96. An α_1-adrenergic receptor antagonist used for hypertension

97. Use of this compound might be expected to specifically inhibit the release of insulin

Questions 98–102:

    A. Propranolol
    B. Haloperidol
    C. Chlorpromazine
    D. Ergonovine
    E. Pindolol

98. A nonspecific β-adrenergic blocking agent with intrinsic sympathomimetic activity

99. This compound possesses significant membrane-stabilizing effects

100. This neuroleptic compound blocks dopamine receptors specifically

101. This alkaloid causes contraction of uterine smooth muscle

102. This agent has been shown to prevent recurrence of myocardial infarction and to decrease mortality

Questions 103–107:

    A. Ganglionic blocking agent
    B. β-Adrenergic blocking agent
    C. α-Adrenergic blocking agent
    D. Neuronal blocking agent
    E. Muscarinic blocking agent

103. Trimethaphan

104. Metyrosine

105. Metoprolol

106. Bretylium

107. Tolazoline

Questions 108–110:

    A. Neostigmine
    B. Cocaine
    C. Tranylcypromine
    D. Propranolol
    E. Pindolol

108. Administration of this local anesthetic compound would potentiate the action of exogenously administered epinephrine

109. A side effect might be excessive salivation

110. Use of this agent must be discontinued slowly

Questions 111–113:

    A. Tetraethylammonium (TEA)
    B. Dimethylphenylpiperazinium (DMPP)
    C. Hexamethonium
    D. Decamethonium
    E. Hemicholinium

111. An activator of nicotinic$_1$ receptors

112. A bisquarternary compound that produces blockade of nicotinic$_2$ receptors

113. Inhibits the high-affinity choline uptake system

Questions 114–119:

    A. Norepinephrine to epinephrine
    B. Dopamine to norepinephrine
    C. Dopa to dopamine
    D. Tyrosine to dopa
    E. Dopa to epinephrine

114. The rate-limiting step in catecholamine synthesis

115. The step in catecholamine synthesis that takes place within the granule

116. This step in the synthesis of biogenic amines takes place in the adrenal medulla and is a methyltransferase reaction

117. This step is a decarboxylation reaction

118. The antihypertensive, α-methyldopa, will substitute for the substrate at this step

119. Catecholamines are feedback inhibitors of this step

Questions 120 – 125:

    A. Acetylcholine
    B. Carbachol
    C. Bethanechol
    D. Methacholine
    E. Choline

120. Agent which is predominately used therapeutically for its cardiovascular effects

121. Resistant to inhibition by atropine and not hydrolyzed by cholinesterases

122. Not employed therapeutically because of its rapid hydrolysis and lack of specificity

123. Used for urinary retention

124. Used in ophthalmology

125. The agent with the greatest possibility of causing ganglionic stimulation upon administration

Questions 126 – 130:

    A. Muscarinic agonists
    B. Anticholinergic agents
    C. Ganglionic blocking drugs
    D. Nicotinic agonists
    E. Nicotinic antagonists

126. Contraindications include asthma, coronary insufficiency, and peptic ulcer

127. Signs of toxicity may include hot dry skin and delirium

128. Stimulates both skeletal muscle and ganglionic sites

129. Ipratropium

130. Belladonna alkaloids

Questions 131–134:

    A. Muscarinic$_1$ (M$_1$)
    B. Muscarinic$_2$ (M$_2$)
    C. Nicotinic$_1$ (N$_1$)
    D. Nicotinic$_2$ (N$_2$)
    E. muscarinic$_1$ (m$_1$)

131. A cloned receptor

132. Provides for alternate transmission through the ganglia

133. Associated with phosphoinositide metabolism

134. Blocked by curare

Questions 135–139:

    A. Guanethidine
    B. Norepinephrine
    C. Reserpine
    D. Ergotamine
    E. Isoproterenol

135. Production of tissue necrosis and sloughing when extravasation occurs during intravenous infusion

136. Cardiac effects with bronchodilating doses

137. Vasoconstricting action on cutaneous blood vessels by action on α-adrenergic receptors

138. Toxic effects of overdose include palpitation, tachycardia, cardiac arrhythmias, flushing of the skin, tremors, nausea, and weakness

139. Useful in the treatment of migraine headaches

Questions 140–142:

    A. Cromolyn
    B. Minoxidil
    C. Timolol
    D. Methyldopa
    E. Propranolol

140. Useful in the prevention of migraine headaches

141. Useful as a prophylactic treatment to prevent attacks of asthma, but ineffective if the asthmatic attack is occurring

142. Side actions and toxic effects include fluid retention, excessive hair growth on the face and back, and pericardial effusion

Questions 143–145:

    A. Pilocarpine
    B. Mecamylamine
    C. Timolol
    D. Metoprolol
    E. Clonidine

143. A nonselective β-adrenergic antagonist useful in the treatment of glaucoma

144. Useful in treatment of glaucoma; drug causes miosis and spasm of the ciliary muscles

145. Useful in treating hypertension due to its CNS effects

Questions 146–148:

    A. Albuterol
    B. Neostigmine
    C. Tyramine
    D. Phentolamine
    E. Cocaine

146. Blocks amine uptake mechanism of neuronal membrane

147. Indirect-acting sympathomimetic amine

148. Effective in the treatment of bronchial asthma

Questions 149-151:

    A. Methoxamine
    B. Ephedrine
    C. Scopolamine
    D. Theophylline
    E. Phentolamine

149. Produces an increase in arterial blood pressure devoid of direct cardiac stimulation

150. Its peripheral, but not its central, actions are reduced by guanethidine

151. Phosphodiesterase inhibitor used in the treatment of asthma

Questions 152 and 153: In Figure 2, the blood pressure graphic record obtained from a dog anesthetized with pentobarbital shows the effects of 10 μg/kg of acetylcholine given intravenously at C and at D.

    A. Atropine
    B. Ephedrine
    C. Epinephrine
    D. Phentolamine
    E. Phenylephrine

152. From the preceding list of drugs, select the one given between injections A and B (Figure 2)

153. From the preceding list of drugs, select the one given between injections C and D (Figure 2)

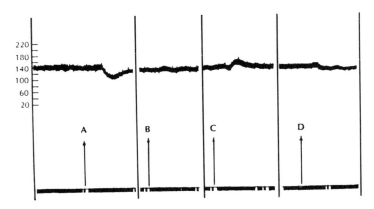

Figure 2 Blood pressure record from dog anesthetized with sodium pentobarbital showing the effects of intravenous injections of acetylcholine 10 μg/kg at A and B and 100 μg/kg at C and D. (Reproduced from Goth A: *Medical Pharmacology*, 11th Ed. St. Louis, CV Mosby, 1984, with permission.)

Questions 154 and 155: The blood pressure graphic record shown in Figure 3 was obtained from a dog anesthetized with pentobarbital.

    A. Atropine
    B. Ephedrine
    C. Epinephrine
    D. Phentolamine
    E. Phenylephrine

154. From the preceding list of drugs, select the one given at A in Figure 3 where time intervals are shown in minutes

155. The drug given at A was injected again at C in the same dosage; from the preceding list of drugs, select the one given at B (Figure 3)

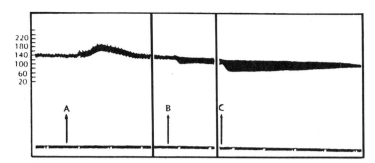

Figure 3 (Reproduced from Goth A: *Medical Pharmacology*, 11th Ed. St. Louis, CV Mosby, 1984, with permission.)

DIRECTIONS (Questions 156–186): Each set of lettered headings below is followed by a list of numbered words or phrases. For each numbered word or phrase select

    A if the item is associated with **A** only
    B if the item is associated with **B** only
    C if the item is associated with both **A** and **B**
    D if the item is associated with neither **A** nor **B**

Questions 156–158:

    A. Muscarinic M_1 receptor
    B. Muscarinic M_2 receptor
    C. Both
    D. Neither

156. Activated by acetylcholine

157. Selectively inhibited by the cholinergic antagonist pirenzepine

158. Possess an ion channel activated by binding of acetylcholine to the α subunit

Questions 159 and 160:

    A. Atropine
    B. Scopolamine
    C. Both
    D. Neither

159. A smaller dose is required to cause mydriasis

160. Most of an oral dose is excreted in the urine

Questions 161–163:

    A. Amphetamine
    B. Ephedrine
    C. Both
    D. Neither

161. Liberates norepinephrine

162. Catecholamine

163. Reduced uterine contractions

Questions 164–166:

    A. Isoproterenol
    B. Metaproterenol
    C. Both
    D. Neither

164. Longer duration of action

165. Agonist primarily for β_2-adrenergic receptors

166. Toxic and side effects include tachycardia, palpitations, nervousness, tremors, and headache

Questions 167 and 168:

    A. Phenoxybenzamine
    B. Phentolamine
    C. Both
    D. Neither

167. Irreversible competitive (nonequilibrium competitive) α-adrenergic antagonist

168. With a large dose, α-adrenergic receptor and histamine receptor blockage occurs

Questions 169–174:

    A. Epinephrine infusion in man (10 μg/min)
    B. Norepinephrine infusion in man (10 μg/min)
    C. Both
    D. Neither

169. Increase in mean arterial blood pressure

170. Increase in heart rate

171. Increase in muscle blood flow

172. Constriction of renal blood vessels

173. Contraction of sphincters of gastrointestinal tract

174. Glycogenolysis

Questions 175 and 176:

    A. Levorotatory isomer
    B. Dextrorotatory isomer
    C. Both
    D. Neither

175. CNS excitatory effects of amphetamine

176. β-blocking activity of propranolol

Questions 177–182:

    A. β_1-adrenergic blocking agent
    B. β_2-adrenergic blocking agent
    C. Both
    D. Neither

177. Labetalol

178. Acebutolol

179. Esmolol

180. Preferable agent for patients with diabetes

181. Type of agent selected for treating hypertension in otherwise healthy patients

182. The type of receptor associated with migraines

Questions 183–186:

    A. α_1 agonists
    B. α_2 agonists
    C. Both
    D. Neither

183. Located at effector sites

184. Inhibition leads to increased output of norepinephrine from nerve endings

185. Preferentially stimulated by circulatory epinephrine

186. Related structurally and fundamentally to muscarinic receptors

DIRECTIONS (Questions 187-199): For each of the questions or incomplete statements below, **one** or **more** of the answers or completions given is correct. Select

   A if only 1, 2, and 3 are correct
   B if only 1 and 3 are correct
   C if only 2 and 4 are correct
   D if only 4 is correct
   E if all are correct

187. It is appropriate under certain circumstances to employ adrenergic amines for
    1. attention-deficit hyperactivity disorder
    2. narcolepsy
    3. allergic reactions
    4. nasal congestion

188. The use of amphetamine-type compounds for obesity
    1. is highly effective
    2. is based on suppression of the lateral hypothalamic feeding center
    3. causes stimulation of the ventromedial satiety center
    4. produces a minor change in metabolic rate

189. The use of orally effective β_2-adrenergic agents
    1. may result in skeletal muscle tremor
    2. has very little risk when used in patients with underlying cardiovascular disease
    3. might be expected to cause "down" regulation of β-receptors
    4. routinely causes a major problem with development of tolerance

	Directions Summarized			
A	**B**	**C**	**D**	**E**
1,2,3	1,3	2,4	4	All are
only	only	only	only	correct

190. In the management of reversible hyperactive airways disease (bronchial asthma)
    1. β_2 agonists provide prompt relief of symptoms
    2. effectiveness of aerosol administration depends on droplets reaching distal airways
    3. both the inhibition of the release of mediators of inflammation and bronchodilation are important components of their action
    4. aerosol therapy limits the β_1 effects as well as the skeletal muscle β_2 effects

191. The use of dobutamine may be complicated by the fact that
    1. dobutamine behaves as a pure β_1-adrenergic agonist
    2. the dextro-isomer is an α_1 antagonist
    3. the levo-isomer is an α_1 agonist
    4. massive increases in peripheral resistance occur with this compound

192. Noncatecholamines
    1. would be expected to have minimal β_2-adrenergic effects
    2. may have direct and indirect actions
    3. are expected to have a longer duration of action when compared with catecholamines
    4. rarely develop tachyphylaxis

193. Structure activity relationships of catecholamines that have clinical relevance include
    1. substitution on the nitrogen leads to increased β-adrenergic activity
    2. the presence of hydroxyl groups at the 3,4 position renders compounds susceptible to COMT
    3. substitution of nonpolar groups on the molecule increases CNS activity
    4. addition of substituents on the α carbon stimulates MAO activity

194. The use of sympathomimetic amines in shock
    1. often requires α_1-specific agents
    2. may be directed at increasing peripheral resistance
    3. may be directed at increasing cardiac contractility
    4. is highly effective in cardiogenic shock

195. Toxic or side effects of reserpine include
    1. untoward effects which are usually those associated with the CNS or the gastrointestinal tract
    2. nightmares
    3. psychic depression
    4. abdominal cramps and diarrhea

196. Which of the following statements is (are) correct concerning Parkinson's disease?
    1. About 95% of orally administered levodopa does not reach the brain as it is metabolized elsewhere into dopamine
    2. Side actions of levodopa include nausea and vomiting early in therapy, and later in some patients cardiac arrhythmias, psychiatric behavior changes, and involuntary movements
    3. Trihexyphenidyl, benztropine, and procyclidine are anticholinergic drugs resembling atropine in their mechanism of action and are useful as supplementary drugs
    4. The phenothiazine and the butyrophenones deplete dopamine from neurones

197. Concerning interference of steps in chemical transmission
    1. guanethidine interferes with release of norepinephrine
    2. reserpine interferes with storage of norepinephrine
    3. methyldopa is metabolized to α-methyl norepinephrine, which by combining with α_2-receptors, inhibits norepinephrine release
    4. pyrogallol interferes with destruction of norepinephrine

Directions Summarized				
A	**B**	**C**	**D**	**E**
1,2,3	1,3	2,4	4	All are
only	only	only	only	correct

198. Which of the following statements is (are) true concerning the use of carbidopa with levodopa?
    1. Carbidopa does not penetrate the blood–brain barrier
    2. Carbidopa permits the use of smaller doses of levodopa
    3. Carbidopa inhibits the decarboxylation of levodopa into dopamine
    4. Carbidopa has been removed from accepted therapy due to its side and toxic effects

199. Concerning the mechanism of action of β-adrenergic drugs
    1. the β agonist acts as a first messenger as it becomes bound to the β-adrenergic receptor
    2. an alteration in intracellular cyclic AMP levels is an integral part of the activation process
    3. the β-receptor is located on the surface and not in the interior of the cell
    4. cyclic AMP is called the second messenger and activates some specific protein kinase

Explanatory Answers

51. C. Prazosin is a unique antihypertensive agent which reduces blood pressure by specifically blocking α_1-receptors. (**Ref.** 1, p. 108; **Ref.** 3, p. 165; **Ref.** 6, p. 188; **Ref.** 8, p. 226; **Ref.** 9, p. 284)

52. C. Nadolol has a half-life of 14 to 18 hours, is a nonselective β-adrenergic blocker, and does not activate β-receptors. (**Ref.** 1, pp. 112–113; **Ref.** 6, pp. 194, 199–200; **Ref.** 8, pp. 234–235)

53. D. Noncatecholamines are resistant to enzymatic inactivation by monoamine oxidase (MAO) or catechol-O-methyltransferase (COMT), leading to oral effectiveness and penetration into the CNS causing stimulation. Much of the action of these compounds is a result of releasing norepinephrine from adrenergic nerve endings. (**Ref.** 6, pp. 164–165; **Ref.** 8, pp. 188–190; **Ref.** 9, p. 138)

54. B. Adrenergic amines can be employed to produce mydriasis without cycloplegia. (**Ref.** 1, p. 99; **Ref.** 6, p. 177; **Ref.** 8, p. 217)

55. C. Both the carbamyl ester and the organophosphate-type anticholinesterase agents covalently bind to the enzyme. Phosphorylation occurs at the esteratic site. Enzyme function is restored over time, with carbamate hydrolysis occurring more rapidly. (**Ref.** 6, pp. 111–113, 121; **Ref.** 8, pp. 132–134; **Ref.** 9, pp. 190–193)

56. D. Bethanechol is useful in treating postoperative, postpartum, and neurogenic urinary retention through its muscarinic agonistic actions on smooth muscle of the urinary bladder. Carbachol is less specific. (**Ref.** 3, p. 103; **Ref.** 6, pp. 104–105; **Ref.** 8, pp. 126, 127; **Ref.** 9, p. 175)

57. C. Amitriptyline, through its cocainelike action, blocks the transport system in the axonal membrane of the adrenergic nerve terminal, resulting in an accumulation of norepinephrine at extracellular sites. (**Ref.** 3, p. 94; **Ref.** 6, p. 416; **Ref.** 8, p. 413)

58. B. The principal mechanism for the termination of adrenergic action appears to be the reuptake of adrenergic neurotransmitter at postganglionic sympathetic nerve terminals. (**Ref.** 1, p. 62; **Ref.** 3, p. 94; **Ref.** 6, p. 86; **Ref.** 8, p. 106; **Ref.** 9, p. 128)

59. E. Epinephrine, 1:1000, is a time-honored drug used in the treatment of acute hypersensitivity reactions to drugs and other allergens. It is also widely used with local anesthetics to delay absorption and prolong anesthesia; however, concentrations of 1:20,000 to 1:100,000 are employed for this purpose. (**Ref.** 1, pp. 102–104; **Ref.** 3, p. 151; **Ref.** 6, pp. 177, 206; **Ref.** 8, pp. 214–218; **Ref.** 9, p. 149)

60. D. The rate-limiting step in the synthesis of the catecholamines is the synthesis of dopa from tyrosine. In parkinsonism, there is an imbalance between dopamine and acetylcholine in the basal ganglia, and treatment with the precursor of dopamine is indicated. (**Ref.** 1, pp. 61–63, 334; **Ref.** 3, pp. 92–93, 123; **Ref.** 6, pp. 82, 474; **Ref.** 8, pp. 102, 463; **Ref.** 9, pp. 127, 501)

61. C. Timolol is a nonselective β-adrenergic antagonist useful in treatment of hypertension and glaucoma. Recently, timolol has been approved for treatment of certain cardiovascular diseases. (**Ref.** 3, pp. 170, 192; **Ref.** 6, p. 200; **Ref.** 8, p. 235; **Ref.** 9, pp. 166, 286)

62. C. All are mechanisms which can influence cholinergic activity. Hemicholinium limits the available choline, thereby restricting or preventing the synthesis and storage of acetylcholine. (**Ref.** 1, p. 68; **Ref.** 3, pp. 86, 91; **Ref.** 6, pp. 91, 215; **Ref.** 8, p. 96; **Ref.** 9, p. 133)

63. B. Botulinus toxin prevents the release of acetylcholine not only in the ganglia but at all cholinergic sites. Death is generally due to respiratory failure. (**Ref.** 1, p. 68; **Ref.** 3, pp. 86, 91, 98; **Ref.** 6, p. 91; **Ref.** 8, p. 97; **Ref.** 9, p. 133)

64. A. Upon intravenous administration of either phenylephrine or methoxamine (both potent vasoconstrictors with little cardiac stimulatory activity), the elicited pressor response initiates vagal reflexes often capable of terminating paroxysmal atrial tachycardia. (**Ref.** 1, p. 103; **Ref.** 3, p. 157; **Ref.** 6, p. 171; **Ref.** 8, p. 216; **Ref.** 9, p. 152)

65. E. By blocking both sympathetic and parasympathetic autonomic ganglia, mecamylamine causes a multitude of effects, some of which are listed in the question. (**Ref.** 1, p. 124; **Ref.** 3, p. 188; **Ref.** 6, pp. 219–220; **Ref.** 9, pp. 294–295)

66. C. Under normal conditions, the amine pump is responsible for the return of the catecholamine to the neuron and for termination of action; very little is metabolized. (**Ref.** 1, pp. 62–64; **Ref.** 3, p. 94; **Ref.** 6, pp. 77, 86; **Ref.** 8, pp. 104, 105, 106; **Ref.** 9, p. 128)

67. E. Bretylium, like guanethidine, has many complex pharmacologic actions on the adrenergic neuron, including release of catecholamines, an antiadrenergic (blocking) effect, and prolongation of the effective refractory period. (**Ref.** 3, pp. 98, 445; **Ref.** 6, p. 207; **Ref.** 8, p. 867; **Ref.** 9, pp. 364–365)

68. C. The release of catecholamines from the adrenal medulla, evoked by stimulation of the splanchnic preganglionic cholinergic fibers or medullary nicotinic cholinergic receptors, is effectively blocked by hexamethonium. (**Ref.** 3, p. 124)

69. D. In the presence of tolerance to epinephrine, corticosteroids or infusion of aminophylline, or both, are indicated and should provide relief. (**Ref.** 1, p. 250; **Ref.** 6, p. 177)

70. D. Since dopamine does not cross the blood–brain barrier efficiently, its precursor, L-dopa, which readily enters the brain, is widely used in the treatment of parkinsonism. (**Ref.** 1, p. 335; **Ref.** 3, p. 122; **Ref.** 6, pp. 475–476; **Ref.** 8, p. 466; **Ref.** 9, p. 502)

71. D. Injurious compounds such as 6-hydroxydopamine (6-OHDA) are readily taken up by the nerve–membrane amine pump and lead to destruction of the sympathetic nerve endings. (**Ref.** 1, p. 68; **Ref.** 3, p. 97; **Ref.** 6, pp. 210–211)

72. D. Atropine, a muscarinic cholinergic blocking agent, blocks all the muscarinic effects of acetylcholine whether they are excitatory or inhibitory. (**Ref.** 1, pp. 126–127; **Ref.** 3, p. 152; **Ref.** 6, p. 132; **Ref.** 9, p. 181)

73. C. Although ergotoxine possesses appreciable α-adrenergic blocking properties, this action is not shared by ergonovine because it lacks the polypeptide side chain necessary for the α-blocking activity in ergot alkaloids. (**Ref. 3**, p. 218; **Ref. 6**, p. 935; **Ref. 8**, p. 142)

74. D. The typical effect of cholinergic agents on the pupil is one of miosis. This effect is caused by a contraction of the circular smooth muscle of the iris, which is under parasympathetic control. (**Ref. 6**, pp. 72–73; **Ref. 8**, pp. 89, 127; **Ref. 9**, pp. 122–123)

75. E. Acetylcholine is the mediator in all ganglia, at skeletal muscle neuromuscular junctions, and at all postganglionic parasympathetic fibers. (**Ref. 1**, p. 60; **Ref. 8**, pp. 97–98; **Ref. 9**, p. 118)

76. C. Uptake$_2$ is an extraneuronal process which may be more important for circulating catecholamines. (**Ref. 8**, p. 105)

77. C. Nicotine, an alkaloid derived from plant sources, causes both acute and chronic toxicity. Its effects may vary considerably depending on the amount taken into the system. (**Ref. 8**, pp. 180–181)

78. A. Norepinephrine is a potent stimulant of α_1-receptors resulting in an increase in peripheral resistance and a reflex decrease in heart rate even though it is a β_1 stimulant. It has little effect on receptors mediating vasodilation (**Ref. 1**, p. 100; **Ref. 8**, pp. 192–193; **Ref. 9**, pp. 141–142)

79. B. Circulating epinephrine does not enter the central nervous system to any extent because it is a polar compound. It does have direct actions causing bronchial smooth muscle relaxation, mydriasis, hyperglycemia, and inhibition of the release of inflammatory mediators. (**Ref. 8**, p. 196)

80. C. The molecular basis of actions involves the interaction of β-receptors with a G protein called G$_s$ resulting in stimulation of adenylyl cyclase while α_2-adrenergic receptors interact with the G protein G$_i$ to inhibit adenylyl cyclase. (**Ref. 8**, p. 111)

81. E. Adrenergic receptor function can be modified by various adaptive changes including phosphorylation, internalization, and modification of portions of the signaling process. (**Ref.** 8, p. 112–113)

82. C. The uterus is influenced by the hormonal background. Most adrenergic agents do not have much therapeutic usefulness with respect to uterine smooth muscle. The exception is β_2 agonists, which inhibit premature labor. (**Ref.** 1, p. 100; **Ref.** 8, p. 196; **Ref.** 9, p. 146)

83. A. The precursor to norepinephrine, dopamine, has effects which vary depending on the concentration employed. At low levels it dilates renal and intestinal vascular beds but as concentrations increase it stimulates β_1-receptors markedly and causes intense α_1 activation. It does not readily cross the blood–brain barrier. (**Ref.** 1, p. 100; **Ref.** 8, p. 200; **Ref.** 9, pp. 147–148)

84. D. The oral use of β_2-adrenergic agonists has significant skeletal muscle tremor as a side effect. While it might be expected that tolerance and/or arrhythmias would occur these are usually not a major clinical problem. Hyperglycemia is produced and insulin may need to be adjusted. (**Ref.** 1, p. 249; **Ref.** 8, p. 206)

85. D. This derivative of atropine is administered by inhalation to treat asthma. Because of its polarity its action tends to remain localized. As an anticholinergic it causes dry mouth. (**Ref.** 8, pp. 159–160; **Ref.** 9, pp. 608–609)

86. E. Metoprolol is a selective β_1-receptor antagonist and should not be confused with the β_2 selective agonist metaproterenol. (**Ref.** 8, pp. 191, 205, 234)

87. A. Agents that block the muscarinic receptor usually have widespread side effects and there has been an active search for selective agents like ipratropium and pirenzepine. Agents currently used cause cycloplegia and do not decrease gastric acid secretion unless high doses are employed. (**Ref.** 1, pp. 85–86; **Ref.** 8, pp. 161–162; **Ref.** 9, pp. 181–182)

88. C. Excess acetylcholine does not occur with ingestion of all mushrooms. It is not the case with *Amanita phalloidies*. *Amanita muscaria* also contains antimuscarinic alkaloids. Pralidoxime is a quaternary compound which does not penetrate the CNS but can reverse organophosphate poisoning if the enzyme has not "aged." (**Ref.** 8, pp. 129, 141)

89. E. By virtue of their structural chemistry, the quaternary amine, neostigmine, does not enter the CNS while the tertiary amine, physostigmine, does. While the term reversible is a relative term, both of these compounds are relatively reversible when compared to organophosphate compounds. (**Ref.** 8, p. 134; **Ref.** 9, pp. 190–192)

90. C. Acetylcholine but not bethanechol will be potentiated by pretreatment with a cholinesterase inhibitor because bethanechol is not a substrate. Hexamethonium blocks at ganglia and scopolamine is a cholinergic muscarinic blocker. (**Ref.** 8, p. 126)

91. B. Pilocarpine is a naturally occurring cholinomimetric alkaloid which will activate muscarinic sites inducing contraction of airways and the precipitation of an asthmatic episode. (**Ref.** 8, pp. 128–129; **Ref.** 9, p. 177; **Ref.** 2, p. 177)

92. B. Cholinergic agonists delay A–V conduction (increase conduction time) and inhibit the SA node. They would be additive with the indirect effects of digitalis and would have a negative inotropic action. (**Ref.** 1, p. 73; **Ref.** 8, p. 125; **Ref.** 9, p. 173)

93. D. It is important to know the predominant tone at various effector sites when attempting to predict the action of a drug that blocks the ganglia. The iris is usually partially contracted. Blocking this effect leads to mydriasis. (**Ref.** 1, pp. 89–91; **Ref.** 8, p. 183; **Ref.** 9, pp. 206–207)

94. C. While phenoxybenzamine is a nonequilibrium α-adrenergic blocking agent it will also block muscarinic, histaminic, and serotonergic receptors. (**Ref.** 1, pp. 107–108; **Ref.** 8, pp. 221, 224; **Ref.** 2, p. 159)

95. E. Yohimbine is an alkaloid which has interest because of its specific α_2-adrenergic blocking activity. (**Ref.** 1, p. 108; **Ref.** 8, p. 221)

96. B. The discovery of the α_1 and α_2 subtypes of adrenergic receptors has lead to the development of specific antagonists and revitalized the use of α blockers for the treatment of hypertension. (**Ref.** 1, p. 108; **Ref.** 8, p. 221; **Ref.** 9, pp. 157–158)

97. E. Any compound that blocks α_2-adrenergic receptors has the potential to inhibit insulin release, but yohimbine, as a specific antagonist, would be expected to have this action. (**Ref.** 8, p. 221; **Ref.** 9, p. 132)

98. E. Propranolol and pindolol are both nonspecific but only pindolol stimulates receptors and may be preferred in patients with limited cardiac function. (**Ref.** 1, p. 112; **Ref.** 8, pp. 229, 235; **Ref.** 9, p. 165)

99. A. Propranolol in high concentrations will stabilize membranes (quinidinelike effect). The clinical significance of this effect is not known since the antiarrhythmic action is related to β-blocking activity. (**Ref.** 1, pp. 112–113; **Ref.** 8, p. 231; **Ref.** 9, p. 165)

100. B. Haloperidol is a specific blocker of dopamine receptors in the renal vascular beds. (**Ref.** 8, p. 229)

101. D. Ergonovine is one of the ergot alkaloids which is useful in treatment of postpartum hemorrhage. Ergotamine is useful for treatment of migraine headaches. (**Ref.** 1, p. 212; **Ref.** 8, p. 228; **Ref.** 9, p. 855)

102. A. Timolol, metoprolol, and propranolol have been shown to be effective, if given after a myocardial infarction, in improving mortality statistics and in preventing recurrence by a mechanism which is not understood. (**Ref.** 1, p. 114; **Ref.** 8, p. 240)

103. A. Trimethaphon is a ganglionic blocking agent with a short duration of action which is used to produce controlled hypotension. (**Ref.** 1, p. 125; **Ref.** 8, p. 184; **Ref.** 9, p. 207)

104. D. Tyrosine hydroxylase, located in the neuronal side of the adrenergic neuron, is inhibited by metyrosine. (**Ref.** 1, p. 68; **Ref.** 8, p. 796; **Ref.** 9, p. 293)

105. B. Specific β_1 antagonism of a competitive nature is produced by metoprolol. (**Ref.** 1, p. 112; **Ref.** 8, p. 234; **Ref.** 9, pp. 165–166)

106. D. The compound bretylium has local anesthetic activity. It accumulates in adrenergic nerve endings, releases catecholamines, and then prevents the release of norepinephrine. (**Ref.** 1, p. 179; **Ref.** 8, p. 866; **Ref.** 9, p. 364)

107. C. Phentolamine and tolazoline are competitive nonspecific α-adrenergic blocking agents. (**Ref.** 1, pp. 106–107; **Ref.** 8, p. 225; **Ref.** 9, p. 160)

108. B. Compounds that interfere with the uptake mechanism responsible for terminating the response to catecholamines potentiate exogenously administered amines. Tranylcypromine would also potentiate the response by inhibiting metabolism but it is not a local anesthetic. (**Ref.** 1, p. 68; **Ref.** 8, p. 116; **Ref.** 9, p. 436)

109. A. Cholinesterase inhibitors are not specific and increased salivation may be bothersome. (**Ref.** 1, p. 81; **Ref.** 8, p. 138; **Ref.** 9, p. 195)

110. D. Propranolol administration will result in an increased sensitivity to adrenergic amines, thus the drug must be removed slowly to allow the body to readjust. This does not occur with pindolol. (**Ref.** 8, p. 238)

111. B. DMPP will stimulate nicotinic receptors. (**Ref.** 8, pp. 115, 181)

112. D. TEA is not a bisquarternary compound. Hexamethonium and decamethonium block at ganglia (nicotinic$_1$) and skeletal muscle (nicotinic$_2$), respectively. (**Ref.** 8, p. 115)

113. E. HC-3, which is one of the hemicholiniums, alters cholinergic function by inhibiting choline uptake, which is necessary for the synthesis of acetylcholine. (**Ref.** 8, p. 113)

114. D. The hydroxylation of tyrosine to dihydroxyphenylalanine (dopa) is the rate-limiting step. (**Ref.** 8, p. 102; **Ref.** 9, p. 127)

115. B. Conversion of dopamine to norepinephrine takes place in the granule. (**Ref.** 8, p. 104; **Ref.** 2, p. 128)

116. A. Conversion of norepinephrine to epinephrine consists of adding a methyl group to the nitrogen. (**Ref.** 1, pp. 62–63; **Ref.** 8, p. 104; **Ref.** 9, p. 127)

117. C. The conversion of an amino acid, dihydroxyphenylalanine, to an amine involves 1-aromatic amino acid decarboxylase. (**Ref.** 8, p. 102; **Ref.** 9, p. 127)

118. C. α-methyldopa is converted to α-methyldopamine and then to α-methylnorepinephrine. (**Ref.** 8, p. 102; **Ref.** 9, p. 294)

119. D. Catecholamines will inhibit the action of tyrosine hydroxylase. (**Ref.** 8, p. 102)

120. D. This agent has selectivity for muscarinic versus nicotinic receptors and is hydrolyzed at a slower rate by acetylcholinesterase than acetylcholine. It is resistant to nonspecific cholinesterase. (**Ref.** 1, p. 74; **Ref.** 8, p. 123; **Ref.** 9, p. 174)

121. B. Primary action is on the intestine and on the urinary bladder. (**Ref.** 1, p. 72; **Ref.** 8, p. 124; **Ref.** 9, p. 175)

122. A. The neurotransmitter has virtually no therapeutic use. (**Ref.** 1, p. 72; **Ref.** 8, p. 122; **Ref.** 9, p. 174)

123. C. Bethanechol is the only agent routinely used for urinary retention and urinary bladder disorders. (**Ref.** 8, p. 127; **Ref.** 9, p. 175)

124. B. The use of carbachol for glaucoma is effective in patients who have become resistant to pilocarpine or physostigmine. (**Ref.** 8, p. 127; **Ref.** 9, p. 175)

125. B. Carbachol has the greatest nicotinic$_1$ activity. (**Ref. 8,** p. 124; **Ref. 9,** p. 175)

126. A. Agents that activate the muscarinic receptor may produce untoward effects in patients with any of the three underlying conditions. (**Ref. 1,** p. 89; **Ref. 8,** p. 126; **Ref. 9,** p. 176)

127. B. Intoxication with atropine also includes a rapid/weak pulse, flushed skin scarlet color, widely dilated pupils, and ataxia. (**Ref. 1,** p. 89; **Ref. 8,** p. 158; **Ref. 9,** p. 186)

128. C. Ganglionic stimulants such as nicotine do not show specificity for nicotinic receptors. (**Ref. 8,** p. 180; **Ref. 9,** pp. 203–204)

129. B. Ipratropium is a quaternary ammonium compound which has selectivity by virtue of its lack of absorption when used locally for inhibition of bronchoconstriction. (**Ref. 1,** p. 250; **Ref. 8,** p. 159; **Ref. 9,** pp. 608–609)

130. B. Agents that block muscarinic receptors are contained in a large number of plants including deadly nightshade, Jimson weed, and henbane. (**Ref. 1,** p. 83; **Ref. 8,** p. 151; **Ref. 9,** p. 178)

131. E. Investigators do not adhere to this convention currently, but the use of lower case letters indicated a cloned receptor. (**Ref. 8,** p. 101)

132. A. Muscarinic$_1$ receptors, which are blockable by atropine, are present in the ganglia. (**Ref. 8,** p. 152)

133. B. Activation of Muscarinic$_2$ receptors causes hydrolysis of polyphosphoinositides and the movement of calcium ion. (**Ref. 8,** p. 153)

134. D. Nicotinic$_2$ receptors located on skeletal muscle neuromuscular junction are blocked by tubocurarine. (**Ref. 8,** p. 170; **Ref. 9,** p. 214)

135. B. In contrast to norepinephrine, isoproterenol possesses only β-receptor stimulatory action and, therefore, does not provoke the α-mediated vasoconstriction produced by norepinephrine resulting in necrosis. (**Ref.** 1, p. 100; **Ref.** 8, p. 201; **Ref.** 9, p. 145)

136. E. Toxic effects with isoproterenol are uncommon and less likely to occur than with epinephrine, but patients should be cautioned against excessive number of inhalations from the inhaler as ventricular fibrillation and death have occurred. (**Ref.** 3, p. 158; **Ref.** 6, p. 161; **Ref.** 8, p. 202; **Ref.** 2, p. 145)

137. B. In contrast to norepinephrine, isoproterenol possesses only β-receptor stimulatory action and, therefore, does not provoke the α-mediated vasoconstriction of cutaneous blood vessels produced by norepinephrine. (**Ref.** 1, p. 100; **Ref.** 8, p. 201; **Ref.** 9, p. 145)

138. E. Toxic effects with isoproterenol are uncommon and less likely to occur than with epinephrine, but patients should be cautioned against excessive number of inhalations from the inhaler as ventricular fibrillation and death have occurred. (**Ref.** 3, p. 158; **Ref.** 8, p. 202; **Ref.** 9, p. 145)

139. D. Ergotamine, when given as early as possible during an attack, will be needed in smaller quantities, and will produce better results and fewer side effects. (**Ref.** 6, pp. 938–939; **Ref.** 8, pp. 945–946)

140. E. Propranolol, a nonselective β-adrenergic antagonist, is competitive in action and is frequently effective in preventing but not relieving migraine headaches. (**Ref.** 6, pp. 199, 939–940; **Ref.** 8, p. 246; **Ref.** 9, p. 167)

141. A. Cromolyn is administered as a powder by inhalation and inhibits antigen-induced liberation of histamine and leukotrienes. (**Ref.** 1, p. 252; **Ref.** 8, p. 631; **Ref.** 9, p. 609)

142. B. In order to reduce the dose and toxicity of minoxidil, a diuretic and a β-adrenergic blocking drug can be administered with minoxidil. (**Ref.** 3, pp. 182–183; **Ref.** 6, pp. 796–797; **Ref.** 8, pp. 802–803; **Ref.** 9, pp. 278–279)

143. C. Timolol is effective in the treatment of chronic wide-angle glaucoma by decreasing production of aqueous humor. Timolol is a β-adrenergic antagonist. (**Ref.** 1, p. 115; **Ref.** 6, p. 200; **Ref.** 8, pp. 235, 240)

144. A. Pilocarpine has been used for many years in the treatment of chronic simple and secondary glaucoma. It is an alkaloid with muscarinic actions; its actions are similar but more prolonged than those of acetylcholine. (**Ref.** 1, pp. 78–79; **Ref.** 3, pp. 103–104; **Ref.** 6, pp. 106–107; **Ref.** 8, p. 129; **Ref.** 9, p. 177)

145. E. Clonidine initially causes some stimulation of α_2-adrenergic receptors. However, administered orally in small doses, any initial rise in blood pressure is minimal or absent. (**Ref.** 3, p. 189; **Ref.** 6, p. 203; **Ref.** 8, p. 208; **Ref.** 9, pp. 296–297)

146. E. Cocaine competitively antagonizes the uptake of amines by the axonal membrane, apparently by inhibiting the ATP-Na$^+$-dependent uptake mechanism of axonal membrane, whereas reserpine blocks the uptake of amines by the granular membrane, apparently by inhibiting the ATP-Mg-dependent uptake mechanism of the granular membrane. (**Ref.** 6, pp. 84–85; **Ref.** 8, pp. 104–105)

147. C. In contrast to the direct-acting sympathomimetic amines (eg, phenylephrine), the indirect-acting sympathomimetic amines (eg, tyramine) produce their agonistic actions through the release of catecholamines from the adrenergic nerve terminal. (**Ref.** 3, p. 154; **Ref.** 6, p. 164; **Ref.** 8, p. 191; **Ref.** 9, p. 137)

148. A. In contrast to methoxamine, a direct-acting α agonist lacking β-receptor actions, albuterol selectively stimulates β_2-receptors to produce bronchodilation. (**Ref.** 6, p. 173; **Ref.** 8, p. 205; **Ref.** 9, pp. 152–153)

149. A. The direct-acting α-adrenergic agonist methoxamine like phenylephrine lacks significant β-agonistic action, whereas ephedrine, a mixed sympathomimetic agonist, produces both α (vasoconstrictor) and β (vasodilation and cardiac stimulatory) effects. (**Ref.** 1, p. 101; **Ref.** 3, pp. 154–156; **Ref.** 6, p. 171; **Ref.** 8, pp. 207, 213–214; **Ref.** 9, pp. 152–153)

150. B. Guanethidine, a peripheral catecholamine depletor, will decrease the peripheral effects of the mixed-acting sympathomimetic amine ephedrine, but will not decrease the central effects of ephedrine since guanethidine penetrates the CNS very poorly. (**Ref.** 3, pp. 154–155, 186; **Ref.** 6, pp. 169–170, 205; **Ref.** 8, pp. 213, 794)

151. D. Theophylline, in contrast to β-adrenergic agonists, produces bronchodilation through three postulated mechanisms: (1) inhibition of phosphodiesterase, (2) translocation of calcium ion, and (3) adenosine receptor antagonism. (**Ref.** 1, pp. 245–246; **Ref.** 3, p. 512; **Ref.** 6, p. 594; **Ref.** 8, p. 623; **Ref.** 9, p. 602)

152. A. The belladonna alkaloids are competitive antagonists to the muscarinic actions of acetylcholine and can prevent the fall in blood pressure from a previously effective dose of acetylcholine. (**Ref.** 1, p. 86; **Ref.** 6, p. 132; **Ref.** 8, p. 155)

153. D. The α-adrenergic blocking drug, phentolamine, competitively antagonizes the blood pressure rise caused by the nicotinic action of the larger dose of acetylcholine. (**Ref.** 6, p. 171; **Ref.** 8, p. 124; **Ref.** 9, p. 174)

154. C. The increased blood pressure resulting from epinephrine administration is shorter in duration than with ephedrine or phenylephrine. With epinephrine, the heart rate is usually increased unless the dose is very large; with phenylephrine, reflex bradycardia occurs because it stimulates only α-adrenergic receptors. (**Ref.** 1, pp. 100–101; **Ref.** 3, pp. 146, 155–157; **Ref.** 6, pp. 169–171; **Ref.** 8, pp. 192, 207; **Ref.** 9, pp. 142, 152)

155. D. Phentolamine is an equilibrium-competitive α-adrenergic antagonist, with a quicker and shorter duration of action than the haloalkylamines. The immediate effect is reduced vasoconstriction and some fall in blood pressure; repeating the administration of epinephrine elicits only β-adrenergic effects. (**Ref.** 1, pp. 106, 109; **Ref.** 3, pp. 163–164; **Ref.** 6, pp. 183–185; **Ref.** 8, p. 223; **Ref.** 9, p. 147)

156. C. Both subtypes of muscarinic receptors are activated by the endogenous neurotransmitter acetylcholine. (**Ref.** 1, p. 83; **Ref.** 3, p. 178; **Ref.** 6, pp. 106, 132, 248; **Ref.** 8, pp. 99, 101)

157. A. The main locations of M_1 receptors, which are identified by preferential binding of pirenzepine, are in the hippocampus, cerebral cortex, and ganglia and they stimulate gastric acid secretion while M_2 receptors are in the gut, heart, and cerebellum. (**Ref.** 1, p. 83; **Ref.** 3, p. 121; **Ref.** 6, pp. 94, 132; **Ref.** 8, p. 101; **Ref.** 9, p. 178)

158. D. The ion channel is a property of the nicotinic$_2$ receptor. (**Ref.** 6, pp. 224, 225; **Ref.** 8, pp. 99, 168)

159. B. The usual systemic dose (0.6 mg) of atropine produces effects on the eyes, but this quantity of scopolamine causes mydriasis and cycloplegia. (**Ref.** 6, pp. 133–134; **Ref.** 8, p. 154; **Ref.** 9, p. 182)

160. A. The larger portion of atropine is excreted in the urine, but only about 1% of the dose of scopolamine is excreted by the kidneys. (**Ref.** 6, p. 137; **Ref.** 8, p. 157)

161. C. Both drugs have indirect action and liberate norepinephrine. (**Ref.** 1, p. 101; **Ref.** 3, p. 154; **Ref.** 6, pp. 166, 169; **Ref.** 8, pp. 191, 213; **Ref.** 9, p. 153)

162. D. Ephedrine and amphetamine have no hydroxyl group on the benzene ring and are not catecholamines. (**Ref.** 1, p. 97; **Ref.** 3, pp. 155, 157; **Ref.** 6, p. 149; **Ref.** 8, p. 189; **Ref.** 9, p. 151)

163. B. Ephedrine reduces uterine contractions, whereas amphetamine usually increases uterine tone. β_2 agonists are employed for termination of premature labor. (**Ref.** 6, pp. 166, 169, 173–174, 942; **Ref.** 8, pp. 210, 213, 949)

164. B. Metaproterenol inhalation provides relief from asthma from 1 to 5 hours due to bronchiole muscular relaxation. The improved respiratory function with isoproterenol inhalation is shorter in duration. (**Ref.** 1, pp. 248–249; **Ref.** 3, p. 158; **Ref.** 6, pp. 172, 176–177; **Ref.** 8, pp. 201, 204)

165. B. Metaproterenol, albuterol, and terbutaline are selective for β_2-receptors. Each has some influence on β_1-receptors. They are used principally to relax bronchioles in asthmatic attacks. (**Ref.** 1, pp. 248–249; **Ref.** 3, pp. 510–511; **Ref.** 6, pp. 172–173; **Ref.** 8, pp. 206–207)

166. C. These are characteristic symptoms of either an overdose or hypersensitivity to sympathomimetic drugs, particularly the β-adrenergic drugs. (**Ref.** 6, pp. 172–173; **Ref.** 8, pp. 206–207; **Ref.** 9, pp. 607–608)

167. A. Phenoxybenzamine is competitive with norepinephrine and other α-adrenergic agonists. It then becomes covalently bound to the receptor and ceases to be reversible; it is now nonequilibrium or irreversible. (**Ref.** 1, p. 107; **Ref.** 3, pp. 163–164; **Ref.** 6, p. 183; **Ref.** 8, p. 224; **Ref.** 9, p. 159)

168. A. Phenoxybenzamine in larger doses blocks acetylcholine, histamine, and serotonin; usual doses of phentolamine primarily block α-adrenergic receptors. (**Ref.** 6, p. 185; **Ref.** 8, p. 224; **Ref.** 9, pp. 158, 160)

169. B. The mean blood pressure effects of epinephrine and norepinephrine reflect their activities at various vascular beds. Norepinephrine induces widespread vasoconstriction (α-receptor stimulation), whereas epinephrine produces constriction of some vascular beds (α-receptor stimulation) and dilation of others (β_2-receptor stimulation). The differences between epinephrine and norepinephrine tend to disappear when they are injected in large doses. (**Ref.** 1, p. 98; **Ref.** 3, p. 148; **Ref.** 6, pp. 152–153; **Ref.** 8, p. 193; **Ref.** 2, p. 141)

170. A. In contrast to norepinephrine infusion, epinephrine at this dose does not significantly elevate blood pressure and activate compensatory reflexes; therefore, it does not antagonize appreciably the direct cardiac actions of epinephrine. The differences between epinephrine and norepinephrine tend to disappear when they are injected in large doses. (**Ref.** 1, p. 98; **Ref.** 3, p. 148; **Ref.** 6, pp. 152–153; **Ref.** 8, p. 193; **Ref.** 9, p. 141)

171. A. Because β_2-receptors are sensitive to much lower concentrations of epinephrine than are the α-receptors, the vasculature of skeletal muscles is dilated by low doses of epinephrine, but constricted by low doses of norepinephrine. The differences between epinephrine and norepinephrine tend to disappear when they are injected in large doses. **(Ref.** 1, p. 97; **Ref.** 3, p. 146; **Ref.** 6, p. 153; **Ref.** 8, p. 190; **Ref.** 9, p. 142)

172. C. α-Adrenergic receptors predominate in the kidney. Both drugs constrict vessels in the kidneys and, at this rate of infusion, reduce blood flow. **(Ref.** 6, p. 153; **Ref.** 8, pp. 89, 194; **Ref.** 9, p. 142)

173. C. The gastrointestinal tract contains both types of adrenergic receptors, but the sphincter contains only the α type. **(Ref.** 6, p. 72; **Ref.** 8, p. 89)

174. A. The presence of β-adrenergic receptors in skeletal muscles and liver brings about glycogenolysis with infusions of epinephrine. However, larger amounts of norepinephrine cause glycogenolysis in the liver. **(Ref.** 1, p. 100; **Ref.** 3, p. 150; **Ref.** 6, pp. 73, 156, 159; **Ref.** 8, pp. 196, 199; **Ref.** 9, p. 146)

175. B. Although both forms of amphetamine possess CNS stimulatory properties, the D-isomer is three to four times as potent as the L-isomer. **(Ref.** 3, p. 159; **Ref.** 6, p. 151; **Ref.** 8, p. 24; **Ref.** 9, p. 153)

176. A. The D-isomer of propranolol has less than 1% of the potency of the L-isomer in blocking β-adrenergic receptors. For most drugs, the L-isomer is more potent on the circulatory system than is the D-isomer. **(Ref.** 3, p. 168; **Ref.** 8, pp. 233–234; **Ref.** 9, p. 164)

177. C. The unique feature of labetalol is that it blocks both β-receptors and also blocks the α_1-adrenergic receptors. **(Ref.** 8, p. 234)

178. A. This is an example of a β_1-adrenergic antagonist. It also has membrane stabilizing activity. **(Ref.** 8, p. 234)

179. A. The duration of esmolol is approximately 10 minutes. Most agents have a plasma half-life of 3 hours. (**Ref.** 8, p. 234)

180. A. β_1-Antagonists such as metoprolol are preferred, since β_2-receptor activation leads to increased insulin release, a process which should not be inhibited in patients with diabetes. (**Ref.** 8, pp. 90, 240)

181. C. The efficiency of most agents is equivalent if no underlying disease process exists. (**Ref.** 8, p. 240)

182. D. Metoprolol (specific), propranolol (nonspecific), and timolol (nonspecific) have all been shown to be effective for migraines. (**Ref.** 8, p. 240)

183. C. α_2-Receptors were once thought to be located only on the adrenergic nerve ending. This is a major functional site but they are also located on effector sites as are α_1-receptors. (**Ref.** 8, p. 110)

184. B. α_2-Receptors inhibit norepinephrine release. Therefore the use of an α_2 or a nonspecific α antagonist increases norepinephrine release. (**Ref.** 8, p. 223)

185. B. It is known that α_2-receptors are activated by both epinephrine and norepinephrine but circulatory epinephrine is thought to preferentially stimulate postsynaptic α_2-receptors. (**Ref.** 8, p. 223)

186. C. Both α_1- and α_2-receptors appear to be related to muscarinic receptors. (**Ref.** 8, p. 110)

187. E. The adrenergic amines are employed therapeutically for both central and peripheral actions. (**Ref.** 1, pp. 103–104; **Ref.** 8, pp. 216–217; **Ref.** 9, pp. 149, 153–154)

188. C. Amphetamines suppress feeding and cause weight loss due to decreased food intake; however, this effect is not sustained due to the rapid development of tolerance in humans. There is no major effect on metabolism. (**Ref.** 8, p. 211)

189. B. Adverse effects of β_2-adrenergic amines include skeletal muscle tremor and cardiac arrhythmias in patients with underlying cardiac disease. While tolerance and down regulation of receptors occurs it is usually not a major problem in patients who adhere to dosing regimens. (**Ref.** 1, pp. 607, 608; **Ref.** 8, p. 206; **Ref.** 9, p. 153)

190. E. Important principles of using β_2-specific agonists include proper administration of the aerosol, to reach the site of action, and to limit adverse systemic effects. (**Ref.** 1, p. 249; **Ref.** 8, p. 204; **Ref.** 9, p. 607)

191. A. Dobutamine is a unique compound that acts by stimulating β_1-receptors in the heart; however, its isomers have opposing effects on α-receptors resulting in a cancellation of the effects on peripheral resistance. (**Ref.** 8, p. 202)

192. A. The lack of the 3-hydroxy group makes noncatecholamines resistant to COMT and hence longer acting. Some of these agents have direct actions, ie, phenylephrine, but others depend on indirect release of norepinephrine (lacks β_2 activity) from nerve endings and thus tachyphylaxis may occur. (**Ref.** 1, p. 101; **Ref.** 8, p. 191; **Ref.** 9, p. 149)

193. A. Basic concepts often include a knowledge of the chemical structure of the compound which allows prediction of clinical usefulness. Substitutions on the nitrogen increase β-receptor activity, while substitutions on the β carbon or the hydroxyl groups increase resistance to metabolic inactivation by MAO and COMT, respectively. Catecholamines do not cross the blood–brain barrier to any extent but increasing lipophilic groups leads to CNS activity. (**Ref.** 1, p. 97; **Ref.** 8, p. 188; **Ref.** 9, pp. 138–139)

194. A. Treatment of shock requires a determination of the appropriate agents. Agents that increase peripheral resistance (α_1 agonists) or cardiac contractility (β_1 agents or dobutamine) may be most appropriate. Adrenergic amines are usually not beneficial in cardiogenic shock. (**Ref.** 1, pp. 102–103; **Ref.** 8, pp. 214–215; **Ref.** 9, p. 152)

195. E. Undesirable side effects may require discontinuing reserpine in some hypertensive patients. It should not be given to patients with a history of peptic ulcer or depressive episodes. (**Ref.** 1, p. 128; **Ref.** 6, p. 209; **Ref.** 8, p. 796; **Ref.** 9, p. 292)

196. A. Anticholinergic drugs are now considered supplemental drugs for the treatment of Parkinson's disease. Amantadine (an antiviral agent) and ergolines (bromocriptine) have been used because they release dopamine and exert dopaminergic activation, respectively. Phenothiazines are considered receptor blockers. (**Ref.** 6, pp. 143, 475–476, 478, 480, 483–484; **Ref.** 8, pp. 468–469, 475–476, 479)

197. E. Additional types of interference with adrenergic nerves are tricyclic antidepressants, which inhibit neuronal transport, and the α- and β-adrenergic blockers, which block combination of transmitters with receptors. (**Ref.** 6, pp. 95, 204, 208; **Ref.** 8, pp. 103, 116, 794)

198. A. Carbidopa seems to be free of side action and toxic effects in the recommended doses. Currently, tablets containing 10 or 25 mg of carbidopa and 100 mg of levodopa and tablets containing 25 mg of carbidopa and 250 mg of levodopa, or carbidopa alone, are available. (**Ref.** 3, p. 123; **Ref.** 8, p. 471; **Ref.** 9, p. 505)

199. E. Current studies indicate that the second messenger is also involved in the action of other neurotransmitters and of hormones. (**Ref.** 6, pp. 37–38, 88–89, 148; **Ref.** 8, pp. 38–40, 109, 148; **Ref.** 9, pp. 11, 139–141)

4 Drugs Affecting the Cardiovascular System

DIRECTIONS (Questions 200–226): Each of the questions or incomplete statements below is followed by five suggested answers or completions. Select the **one** that is best in each case.

200. The preferred agent for hypertensive emergencies is
    A. diazoxide
    B. sodium nitroprusside
    C. propranolol
    D. reserpine
    E. clonidine

201. All of the following statements about nitroglycerin are true EXCEPT
    A. nitrates relax the smooth muscles of both arteries and veins
    B. low levels of nitroglycerin cause a greater venodilation than arteriodilation
    C. the primary action of nitroglycerin is to increase coronary blood flow
    D. nitrates appear to cause a redistribution of coronary blood flow
    E. nitroglycerin has a greater relaxant effect on large versus small coronary arteries

202. Digoxin would be the choice for long-term treatment of congestive heart failure resulting from
   A. essential hypertension
   B. thyrotoxicosis
   C. severe myocardial infarction
   D. anemia
   E. mechanical obstruction

203. The effects of quinidine include
   A. an increase in the force of myocardial contraction
   B. an indirect effect to decrease atrial–ventricular (A–V) conduction time
   C. vasoconstriction
   D. activation of sodium channels
   E. hypertensive episodes

204. Which of the following statements are true regarding the diagrams in Figure 4?
   A. The action of class I antiarrhythmic drugs should be diagrammed as the change occurring between panels B and D
   B. Digitalis would be expected to suppress the type of activity diagrammed in panel A and convert it to panel C-type response
   C. The monophasic action potential shown in panel E could be converted by procainamide to the pattern seen in panel A
   D. Calcium channel blockers act primarily to alter the phase 4 potential shown in panel E
   E. Verapamil restores and stimulates the delayed depolarization diagrammed in panel C

205. In the therapy of congestive heart failure, the most important pharmacologic action of digitalis is its ability to
   A. produce diuresis in edematous patients
   B. reduce venous pressure
   C. increase myocardial contractile force
   D. increase heart rate
   E. decrease pacemaker automaticity in cells of the bundle of His

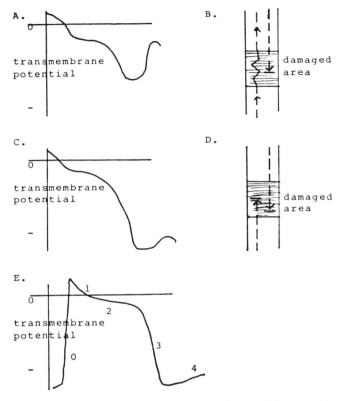

Figure 4 (Composite diagram adapted from Goth A: *Medical Pharmacology*, 11th Ed. St. Louis, CV Mosby, 1984, p. 439; Gilman AG, Goodman LS, Rall TW, Murad F: *Goodman and Gilman's The Pharmacological Basis of Therapeutics*, 7th Ed. New York, Macmillan, 1985, pp. 752–753, with permission.)

206. Of the following cardiac glycosides, which has the clearly superior (larger) therapeutic index?
    A. Ouabain
    B. Digoxin
    C. Digitoxin
    D. Deslanoside
    E. None of the above is superior to the others

207. Digoxin differs from digitoxin in that digoxin
  A. has a longer half-life
  B. is completely absorbed from the gastrointestinal (GI) tract
  C. has a half-life that is more dependent on the adequacy of renal function
  D. is bound extensively to the plasma proteins
  E. is metabolized extensively by the liver

208. When digitalis is given to the typical patient with congestive failure and atrial fibrillation
  A. cardiac output is unchanged
  B. ventricular rate is slowed by both vagal and direct effect
  C. ventricular efficiency is decreased
  D. a decrease in heart rate is a primary effect
  E. none of the above occurs

209. Which of the following statements regarding blood lipids is true?
  A. No convincing data have been published yet to show a high correlation between patients with familial hypercholesterolemia and myocardial infarction
  B. Epinephrine can cause a rise in serum lipids, but chronic administration has no effect on experimental atherosclerosis
  C. Polyunsaturated oils, such as corn oil, will promote fecal excretion of cholesterol
  D. In patients, clofibrate is more effective in lowering plasma triglycerides than plasma cholesterol
  E. Although there are several patterns of hyperlipoproteinemia, therapy is the same for all types

210. Which of the following statements is true concerning cholestyramine?
   A. It inhibits free fatty acid release from adipose tissue
   B. It releases lipoprotein lipase
   C. It is an anion-exchange resin that binds bile acid in the human intestinal lumen
   D. It blocks the final step in the formation of cholesterol in the body
   E. When used in large doses, it decreases serum cholesterol, triglycerides, and phospholipids, possibly via an effect on synthesis

211. Quinidine is either contraindicated or should be used with caution in all of the following EXCEPT
   A. complete A – V block
   B. digitalis intoxication
   C. severe congestive heart failure
   D. atrial fibrillation of recent origin
   E. a history of thrombocytopenic purpura due to previous use of quinidine

212. The syndrome of cinchonism includes all of the following symptoms EXCEPT
   A. tinnitus
   B. delirium
   C. disturbed vision
   D. hypertensive reaction
   E. headache

213. Side effects that might be expected with hydralazine include all of the following EXCEPT
   A. headache
   B. palpitations
   C. A – V block
   D. anginal attacks
   E. acute rheumatoid symptoms

214. Regarding the effects of digitalis on conduction and refractory period, all of the following statements are true EXCEPT

A. A – V nodal conduction is slowed by the vagal effect, but this is opposed by the direct effect
B. the P-R interval of the ECG is prolonged
C. the refractory period of the A – V node is prolonged
D. the refractory period of the ventricle is usually either unchanged or shortened
E. the refractory period of the atrium is usually shortened in humans

215. In the typical patient with congestive heart failure, digitalis would be expected to do all of the following EXCEPT

A. decrease the diastolic heart size
B. increase the cardiac output
C. increase sympathetic activity
D. increase vital capacity
E. decrease blood volume

216. The antihypertensive agent that acts by inhibiting the formation of angiotensin is

A. hydralazine
B. captopril
C. minoxidil
D. propranolol
E. reserpine

217. The effects of digoxin on transmembrane electrograms would be expected to include

A. a decrease in the rate of change of dV/dt in phase 4
B. a lengthening of phase 2 and 3
C. the production of early after-depolarizations
D. an increase in the slope of phase 4
E. an increase in action potential duration

218. The mechanism of action of digitoxin
  A. is different from that of digoxin
  B. depends on the stimulation of Na^+, K^+-ATPase
  C. is due to inhibition of sodium transport
  D. results in increased intracellular sodium which exchanges for calcium
  E. depends on increased levels of intracellular ATP

219. Antiarrhythmic agents would decrease generation arrhythmias by
  A. increasing dV/dt in phase 0
  B. decreasing resting membrane potential
  C. converting bidirectional conduction to unidirectional conduction
  D. altering threshold potential
  E. none of the above

220. In reference to antiarrhythmic drugs, all the following statements are true EXCEPT
  A. class Ic agents are proarrhythmogenic
  B. encainide has been demonstrated to increase the risk of sudden cardiac death
  C. flecainide will effectively prevent unsustained ventricular arrhythmias in patients with a recent myocardial infarction
  D. cimetidine may cause an increase in toxicity of encainide
  E. propafenone may cause a systemic lupus erythematosus (SLE)-like syndrome

221. All of the following statements are true EXCEPT
  A. heparin acts both in vitro and in vivo
  B. coumadin acts in vivo only
  C. heparin may enter the placenta causing internal bleeding
  D. coumadin is considered a vitamin K antagonist
  E. heparin must be administered intravenously

222. The lowering of plasma lipids by lovastatin occurs because it
    A. inhibits HMG coenzyme A (CoA) reductase
    B. binds bile acids
    C. blocks the synthesis of low-density lipoprotein (LDL)
    D. stimulates HMG CoA excretion
    E. none of the above

223. In the reduction of elevated blood pressure all of the following pairings are appropriate EXCEPT
    A. enalapril/acetylcholine esterase inhibitor
    B. methyldopa/α_2 agonist
    C. metyrosine/tyrosine hydroxylase inhibitor
    D. clonidine/α_2 agonist
    E. prazosin/α_1 antagonist

224. Organic nitrates
    A. stimulate cAMP production
    B. inhibit the synthesis of cGMP
    C. result in the formation of NO
    D. block cGMP-dependent protein kinase
    E. lead to phosphorylation of myosin light chain kinase

225. All the following statements are true regarding procainamide EXCEPT
    A. replacement of the nitrogen with a carbon results in procaine
    B. N-acetylprocainamide, a metabolite, has antiarrhythmic action
    C. procainamide may produce thrombocytopenia
    D. an SLE-like syndrome is apt to occur sooner in "slow acetylators" of procainamide
    E. procainamide should be administered with caution to patients with bronchial asthma

226. The compound that must be metabolized to achieve its therapeutic effect is
    A. minoxidil
    B. hydralazine
    C. propranolol
    D. diazoxide
    E. phentolamine

DIRECTIONS (Questions 227–232): This section consists of a clinical situation followed by a series of questions. Study the situation and select the **one** best answer to each question following it.

Questions 227–229: A patient appears in the emergency room with an accelerated ventricular heart rate approaching 190 beats/min. Upon discussion with the spouse it is determined that the patient is taking digoxin along with hydrochlorothiazide and eats large quantities of bananas.

227. The first action taken should be
   A. administration of quinidine
   B. intravenous lidocaine
   C. intravenous potassium
   D. oral procainamide
   E. an intravenous drip of magnesium

228. An important element in the treatment of digitalis intoxication that is often overlooked is
   A. administration of Fab antibody fragments
   B. monitoring the electrocardiogram
   C. determination of serum potassium levels
   D. withdrawal of the cardiac glycoside
   E. administration of potassium

229. In the above case the first step should not be administration of potassium ion because
   A. it could lead to cardiac arrest
   B. potassium is difficult to administer
   C. magnesium is a better choice
   D. automaticity may be increased
   E. A–V block may occur

Questions 230–232: Early in September a female patient arrives at your office complaining of shortness of breath and pounding in the chest. On examination you find that her blood pressure is 140/90, heart rate is 120 beats/min, and no "p" waves are present in the ECG.

230. The decision is to administer digitalis because
  A. congestive heart failure is suspected
  B. it will dilate the airways and improve breathing
  C. the "p" waves need to be restored
  D. the patient has hypertension
  E. cardiac glycosides have minimal effects on the ECG

231. The safest approach to therapy is
  A. digitalization with digoxin
  B. digitalization with digitoxin
  C. intravenous administration of acetyl strophanthidin
  D. administration of maintenance doses of digoxin
  E. administration of maintenance doses of digitoxin

232. The earliest sign of effectiveness would probably be
  A. diuresis
  B. a decrease in heart rate
  C. yellow-green vision
  D. gynecomastia
  E. diarrhea

DIRECTIONS (Questions 233–238): Each group of questions below consists of five lettered headings followed by a list of numbered words, phrases, or statements. For each numbered word, phrase, or statement, select the **one** lettered heading that is most closely associated with it. Each lettered heading may be selected once, more than once, or not at all.

Questions 233–235:

  A. Phenytoin
  B. Papaverine
  C. Digitalis
  D. Reserpine
  E. Propranolol

233. When used as an antagonist to digitalis-induced arrhythmias, can increase the degree of A–V block

234. A drug devoid of negative inotropic effects and is effective in the treatment of ventricular ectopic rhythms

235. Effective in heart failure associated with low cardiac output

Questions 236 – 238:

    A. Digoxin
    B. Cholestyramine
    C. Digitoxin
    D. Quinidine
    E. Nitroglycerin

236. Cardiac glycoside that undergoes extensive hepatic degradation

237. Inhibits vitamin K absorption

238. Increases conductivity of A – V node by blocking the vagus

---

DIRECTIONS (Questions 239 – 268): Each set of lettered headings below is followed by a list of numbered words and phrases. For each numbered word or phrase select
    A if the item is associated with **A** only
    B if the item is associated with **B** only
    C if the item is associated with both **A** and **B**
    D if the item is associated with neither **A** nor **B**

Questions 239 – 241:

    A. Amrinone
    B. Amiodarone
    C. Both
    D. Neither

239. A positive cardiac inotropic agent

240. An antiarrhythmic agent originally developed for angina

241. Use is restricted to a specific group of patients

Questions 242–244:

    A. Atenolol
    B. Labetalol
    C. Both
    D. Neither

242. This antihypertensive compound will inhibit both α_1- and β-receptor function

243. An antihypertensive agent that acts centrally to stimulate α-adrenergic receptors

244. A specific β_1 agonist

Questions 245 and 246:

    A. Warfarin
    B. Heparin
    C. Both
    D. Neither

245. Antagonized by protamine

246. Orally effective

Questions 247–249:

    A. Amiodarone
    B. Disopyramide
    C. Both
    D. Neither

247. Class III antiarrhythmic agent

248. Classed as an Ic agent

249. A fairly high incidence of anticholinergic side effects

Questions 250 and 251:

    A. Tocainide
    B. Bretylium
    C. Both
    D. Neither

250. Major adverse reactions include tremor and gastrointestinal upset

251. Orally effective agent associated with the production of antinuclear antibodies (ANA)

Questions 252–256:

    A. Digoxin
    B. Digitoxin
    C. Both
    D. Neither

252. Longer acting than ouabain (strophanthin)

253. Usually about 75% to 80% of oral dose is absorbed

254. Cardioactive steroid capable of binding to membrane-bound Na^+, K^+-adenosine-triphosphatase (Na^+, K^+-ATPase)

255. Increases cardiac stroke output in the normal heart and in the failing heart

256. Increases force of contraction and the speed of the contractile process in the failing heart

Questions 257–259:

    A. Niacin
    B. Clofibrate
    C. Both
    D. Neither

257. Cause(s) intense cutaneous vasodilation and pruritus

258. Contraindicated in patients with history of peptic ulcer

259. Associated with cholelithiasis

Questions 260–262:

    A. Phenytoin
    B. Propranolol
    C. Both
    D. Neither

260. Increases the effective refractory period (ERP) of the A–V node

261. Overcomes transmission effects of digitalis toxicity, returning it toward normal

262. Cardiac effects including toxic ones are reduced by glucagon

Questions 263–266:

    A. Lidocaine
    B. Quinidine
    C. Both
    D. Neither

263. Bound to α_1-acid glycoprotein

264. Often administered with a preservative or vasoconstrictor

265. In presence of hypokalemia, the antiarrhythmic effects are markedly reduced

266. Effective when administered orally

Questions 267–268:

    A. Digoxin
    B. Quinidine
    C. Both
    D. Neither

267. Electrocardiographic changes in lead 1 produced by this drug (changes are shown in Figure 5)

268. Drug responsible for the change from curve B to curve C in this graph of ventricular end–diastolic volume on the abscissa and ventricular stroke–work on the ordinate where A is normal, B is cardiac failure, and C is cardiac failure after treatment with one of the drugs (Figure 6)

DIRECTIONS (Questions 269–278): For each of the questions or incomplete statements below, **one** or **more** of the answers or completions given is correct. Select
    A if only 1, 2, and 3 are correct
    B if only 1 and 3 are correct
    C if only 2 and 4 are correct
    D if only 4 is correct
    E if all are correct

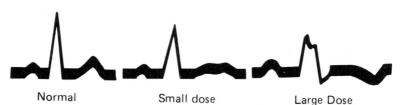

    Normal   Small dose   Large Dose

Figure 5 (Reproduced from Burch GE, Winsor T: *A Primer of Electrocardiography.* Philadelphia, Lea and Febiger, 1960, with permission.)

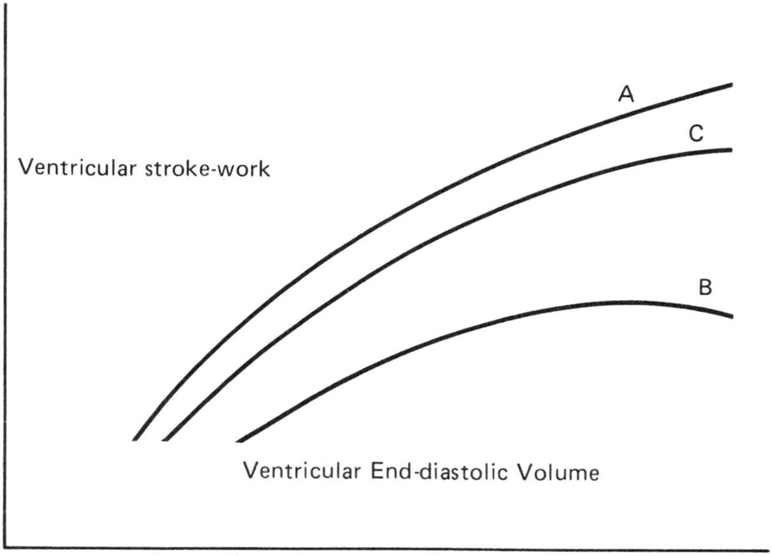

Figure 6

269. Which of the following statements is (are) true concerning calcium channel blockers?
1. Nifedipine produces marked vasodilation
2. Calcium channel blockers are more effective when used with β-adrenergic blockers
3. Verapamil increases blood flow in skeletal muscle vascular beds
4. Diltiazem increases coronary vascular resistance

270. Side effects common to calcium channel blockers include
1. dizziness and flushing
2. worsening of myocardial ischemia
3. tachycardia
4. excessive vasodilation

271. Minoxidil
1. causes arteriovasodilation
2. stimulates renin secretion
3. may cause a marked increase in cardiac output
4. stimulates the growth of hair

		Directions Summarized		
A	**B**	**C**	**D**	**E**
1,2,3	1,3	2,4	4	All are
only	only	only	only	correct

272. The management of angina pectoris includes which of the following as primary agents?
    1. Organic nitrites
    2. Calcium channel blockers
    3. Inhibitors of platelet aggregation
    4. Organic nitrates

273. Administration routes of nitroglycerin for angina pectoris include
    1. transdermal
    2. ointment
    3. sublingual
    4. intravenous

274. The treatment of variant angina
    1. is most effective with nitroglycerin
    2. is ineffective with agents that relieve ergonovine-induced spasm
    3. has been clearly established to be superior when verapamil is utilized
    4. is very effectively managed with calcium channel blockers

275. Concerning the treatment of angina pectoris, which of the following statements is (are) true?
    1. Dipyridamole is a highly effective compound
    2. Dipyridamole probably works by inhibiting adenosine uptake
    3. The actions of dipyridamole are dependent on nitric ion formation
    4. Dipyrimadole is probably most effective in preventing platelet aggregation

276. The use of vasodilators in the treatment of congestive heart failure is based on
  1. the predominant effect of these compounds on venous smooth muscle
  2. an effect of nitroprusside to inhibit cyclic-GMP formation
  3. the development of additional contractile force in the heart
  4. the reduction of cardiac preload and/or afterload

277. Electrocardiographic effects of digitalis include
  1. lengthening of the P-R interval
  2. shortening of the Q-T interval
  3. inversion of the T wave
  4. widening of the QRS complex in Wolf–Parkinson–White (WPW) syndrome

278. Regarding the structure of cardiac glycosides
  1. the aglycone is devoid of action on the heart
  2. the compound possesses sugar molecules as part of its structure
  3. it requires a carboxyl group at position 17 for optimal activity
  4. the unsaturated lactone is an essential component of its structure

Explanatory Answers

200. B. Intravenous administration of sodium nitroprusside will cause rapid vasodilation of arterial and venous vessels. Diazoxide is not useful for all types of emergencies. The other agents are used orally for long-term management. (**Ref.** 1, p. 132; **Ref.** 3, p. 183; **Ref.** 8, p. 810; **Ref.** 9, p. 280)

201. C. The beneficial effect of nitroglycerin is not fully understood but it appears that it increases oxygen supply to the myocardium and, probably most importantly, decreases cardiac work thus reducing oxygen demand. (**Ref.** 1, p. 143; **Ref.** 3, p. 452; **Ref.** 8, p. 766)

202. A. The most common precipitating cause of congestive heart failure is essential hypertension where cardiac output is low. The other four precipitating factors are not effectively managed with cardiac glycosides. (**Ref.** 6, p. 737; **Ref.** 8, pp. 830–831; **Ref.** 9, p. 314)

203. B. Quinidine is a blocker of sodium channels resulting in negative inotropic effects. It also causes vasodilation and may cause hypotensive (quinidine syncope) episodes. Because of its anticholinergic effect A–V conduction may be increased. (**Ref.** 1, p. 172; **Ref.** 3, pp. 437–439; **Ref.** 8, p. 851; **Ref.** 9, p. 341)

204. A. In conduction defect arrhythmias the mechanism of action of class I agents is the conversion of one-way block (retrograde conduction) to two-way block. Digitalis promotes delayed after–depolarization-type of abnormal generation of impulses diagrammed in panel C of Figure 4. Calcium channel blockers alter the slow calcium channel (phase 2). (**Ref.** 1, pp. 168–170; **Ref.** 6, pp. 752–753, 777; **Ref.** 8, p. 845)

205. C. The pharmacodynamic action of cardiac glycosides, to increase the force of myocardial contraction, is well-recognized and has been relied on for treatment of congestive heart failure. This view is being reevaluated. (**Ref.** 3, p. 49; **Ref.** 6, p. 732; **Ref.** 8, pp. 815, 830)

206. E. The qualitative actions of all digitalis compounds are approximately equal and all have approximately the same therapeutic index. (**Ref. 3**, p. 424; **Ref. 8**, p. 832)

207. C. Because it is not readily metabolized but is excreted rapidly, and unchanged in the urine, digoxin has a half-life that is dependent in large measure on the adequacy of renal function. (**Ref. 1**, p. 154; **Ref. 3**, p. 424; **Ref. 6**, pp. 733–735; **Ref. 8**, p. 828; **Ref. 9**, pp. 313–314)

208. B. Digitalis decreases the ventricular rate by prolonging the refractory period of the A–V conduction tissue through both direct and vagal effects. (**Ref. 1**, p. 159; **Ref. 3**, p. 422; **Ref. 6**, pp. 728, 738; **Ref. 8**, p. 820; **Ref. 9**, p. 312)

209. D. Plasma triglyceride concentration is reduced within 5 days of the onset of clofibrate therapy by lowering the levels of very low-density lipoproteins (VLDL). Since a large fall in VLDL may be accompanied by a rise in low-density lipoproteins (LDL), the net effect on cholesterol may be slight. (**Ref. 1**, p. 425; **Ref. 3**, pp. 493, 499; **Ref. 6**, pp. 829, 833, 835–837; **Ref. 8**, pp. 874, 886; **Ref. 9**, pp. 238, 245)

210. C. Cholestyramine is the chloride salt of a quaternary ammonium anion-exchange resin that binds bile acids in the intestine, exchanging them for the chloride ion. (**Ref. 1**, p. 427; **Ref. 3**, p. 500; **Ref. 6**, p. 840; **Ref. 8**, p. 890; **Ref. 9**, pp. 240–241)

211. D. Atrial fibrillation of recent origin is an indication rather than a contraindication for the use of quinidine. (**Ref. 1**, pp. 172–173; **Ref. 6**, pp. 760–762; **Ref. 8**, pp. 854–856; **Ref. 9**, pp. 342, 343)

212. D. Hypotension, which is the result of peripheral vasodilation, is a consistent effect of quinidine overdosage, especially if the drug is given intravenously. (**Ref. 6**, pp. 762, 1044; **Ref. 8**, pp. 855–856, 992–993; **Ref. 9**, p. 343)

213. C. Hydralazine, a direct-acting vascular smooth muscle relaxant, has not been reported to produce A–V block. (**Ref.** 1, p. 132; **Ref.** 3, p. 182; **Ref.** 6, p. 796; **Ref.** 8, p. 800; **Ref.** 9, p. 278)

214. A. The indirect (vagal) and direct effects of digitalis on A–V nodal conduction are synergistic and lead to dose-related depression of A–V conduction. (**Ref.** 1, p. 157; **Ref.** 3, p. 421; **Ref.** 6, p. 725; **Ref.** 8, pp. 820–821; **Ref.** 9, p. 312)

215. C. Digitalis, by improving cardiac and circulatory function, decreases existing high sympathetic activity, which is a compensatory reflex in congestive failure. (**Ref.** 1, p. 158; **Ref.** 6, pp. 731–732; **Ref.** 8, p. 826; **Ref.** 9, pp. 307–310)

216. B. The angiotensin-converting enzyme inhibitors are useful in treating hypertension with minimal side effects. (**Ref.** 8, pp. 806–807; **Ref.** 9, p. 229)

217. D. Cardiac glycosides increase automaticity (phase 4) and shorten refracting period (action potential duration/phase 2 and 3). (**Ref.** 8, p. 819)

218. D. Inhibition of Na^+, K^+-ATPase occurs but it is the exchange of calcium ion which makes contractile calcium available. ATP does not accumulate and all cardiac glycosides act by the same mechanism. (**Ref.** 8, p. 817; **Ref.** 9, p. 311)

219. D. Generation-type arrhythmias can be inhibited by altering threshold (less negative), increasing resting membrane potential, and decreasing automaticity. (**Ref.** 8, p. 840; **Ref.** 9, pp. 336–337)

220. C. The cardiac arrhythmia suppression test (CAST) demonstrated that these new agents should not be used to routinely suppress all arrhythmias. (**Ref.** 8, p. 863; **Ref.** 9, p. 356)

221. C. Intravenous heparin is immediately effective while oral coumadin interferes with clotting factor synthesis. Heparin does not cross into the placenta or into breast milk. (**Ref.** 8, pp. 1314, 1317; **Ref.** 9, pp. 373, 375)

222. A. Lovastatin is an inhibitor of the enzyme that synthesizes cholesterol. Cholestyramine binds bile acids and the synthesis of LDL is not influenced by probucol. (**Ref.** 8, pp. 883, 889, 892; **Ref.** 9, pp. 240, 243 – 244)

223. B. Methyldopa is converted to α-methylnorepinephrine, which is the α_2 agonist that acts centrally. (**Ref.** 8, p. 789; **Ref.** 9, p. 295)

224. C. Organic nitrates and nitrites cause cGMP formation leading to nitric oxide formation and dephosphorylation of myosin. (**Ref.** 8, p. 768; **Ref.** 9, p. 325)

225. C. Quinidine usually produces thrombocytopenia whereas procainamide has a toxic effect of causing SLE-like syndrome. (**Ref.** 8, pp. 856 – 857; **Ref.** 9, pp. 344 – 345)

226. A. Minoxidol is converted to minoxidil N-O sulfate and evidence seems to indicate that it changes membrane permeability to K^+. (**Ref.** 8, p. 801)

227. B. The most effective agent would be lidocaine to control the accelerated ventricular rate. While hypokalemia might be expected due to the use of thiazides, the patient is ingesting food that contains large amounts of potassium ion. (**Ref.** 8, p. 834; **Ref.** 9, p. 317)

228. D. The management of digitalis intoxication includes or may include all of the choices; however, it is often forgotten that administration of the offending agent should cease. (**Ref.** 8, p. 834; **Ref.** 9, p. 317)

229. E. In a patient who has been ingesting potassium-containing food, the levels of potassium should be determined before administration of potassium ion. Serum levels of potassium on the order of 4 mm lead to complete A – V block and potassium is contraindicated. (**Ref.** 6, p. 743; **Ref.** 8, p. 835; **Ref.** 9, p. 317)

230. A. This patient most likely has congestive heart failure and administration of cardiac glycosides will increase vagal tone thus slowing the heart rate as well as improving cardiovascular dynamics. This results in the removal of edema fluid which has accumulated and in improved breathing. (**Ref.** 6, pp. 736–737; **Ref.** 8, pp. 830–831; **Ref.** 9, p. 314)

231. D. This patient is not in severe enough distress to warrant intravenous or rapid administration of cardiac glycosides. It is safer to allow adjustments to occur at a slower rate. Unless other factors warrant a change, digoxin would be preferred. (**Ref.** 1, p. 159; **Ref.** 6, pp. 734–735; **Ref.** 8, p. 829)

232. B. All of the items listed could be an indication of an effect of digitalis, especially toxicity, but the indirect effect of digitalis, which is to increase vagal tone and decrease heart rate, would be noticed first. (**Ref.** 6, pp. 729, 738; **Ref.** 8, pp. 823, 832; **Ref.** 9, p. 316)

233. E. Withdrawal of cardiac sympathetic tone by administration of the β-blocker propranolol accentuates vagal influences on the heart to increase the degree of A–V block. (**Ref.** 6, p. 774; **Ref.** 8, p. 866; **Ref.** 9, p. 361)

234. A. Phenytoin is used to manage both supraventricular and ventricular ectopic rhythms when digitalis is the causative agent. However, lidocaine is usually preferred. (**Ref.** 1, pp. 160, 178; **Ref.** 3, p. 444; **Ref.** 6, pp. 770–771; **Ref.** 8, p. 854; **Ref.** 9, p. 351)

235. C. In contrast to the minor benefits obtained with digitalis in the so-called high-output failures that occur with A–V fistula, thyrotoxicosis, and other conditions, the best results with digitalis cardiac glycosides are obtained in heart failure associated with low cardiac output. (**Ref.** 6, p. 737; **Ref.** 8, pp. 830–831)

236. C. In contrast to digoxin, which is essentially excreted unchanged in the urine, digitoxin undergoes significant hepatic degradation and enterohepatic recirculation, with approximately 25% of the metabolic end products appearing in the feces. The serum half-life of digoxin in humans is 1.5 days, whereas the serum half-life of digitoxin is 5 to 7 days. (**Ref.** 1, p. 154; **Ref.** 8, p. 829; **Ref.** 9, p. 314)

237. B. The anion-exchange resin cholestyramine may interfere via binding with the absorption of fat-soluble vitamins such as K and numerous drugs including the cardiac glycosides. (**Ref.** 1, pp. 411, 427; **Ref.** 3, pp. 500, 749; **Ref.** 8, p. 891)

238. D. Quinidine, through its vagolytic effects, can increase the conductivity of the A–V node. (**Ref.** 1, p. 172; **Ref.** 8, p. 851; **Ref.** 9, p. 341)

239. A. Amrinone, a bipyridine derivative, increases the force of myocardial contraction and is useful in selected cases of congestive heart failure. (**Ref.** 1, p. 158; **Ref.** 3, pp. 431, 433; **Ref.** 6, pp. 743–744; **Ref.** 8, p. 836; **Ref.** 9, p. 320)

240. B. Amiodarone has been used for a wide spectrum of atrial and ventricular arrhythmias. It may cause corneal deposits and a bluish color of the skin. (**Ref.** 1, p. 176; **Ref.** 3, p. 446; **Ref.** 6, pp. 776–777; **Ref.** 8, pp. 867–868; **Ref.** 9, pp. 366–367)

241. C. The use of amiodarone has been restricted to management of life-threatening arrhythmias. Amrinone is useful in selected cases. (**Ref.** 8, p. 868; **Ref.** 9, p. 366)

242. B. Atenolol is β_1-receptor selective, while labetalol inhibits α_1-, β_1-, and β_2-adrenergic receptors. (**Ref.** 3, p. 170; **Ref.** 6, p. 202; **Ref.** 8, p. 236; **Ref.** 9, p. 169)

243. D. The centrally acting α_2-adrenergic agonist is clonidine. Its action is blocked by the α_2-antagonist yohimbine. (**Ref.** 8, p. 208)

244. D. Atenolol is a specific β_1-blocker used for treating hypertension. (**Ref.** 8, p. 237; **Ref.** 9, p. 165)

245. B. If bleeding becomes severe, the use of 1 mg of positively charged protamine will antagonize 100 units of heparin. Mild effects are managed by discontinuing heparin administration. (**Ref.** 6, p. 1344; **Ref.** 8, p. 1317; **Ref.** 9, p. 374)

246. A. The 4-hydroxycoumadin compounds are orally effective anticoagulants, whereas the heparin mucopoly saccharide is not absorbed orally. (**Ref.** 8, pp. 1315, 1319; **Ref.** 9, pp. 373, 375)

247. A. Class III antiarrhythmic drugs include amiodarone and bretylium. These agents are not well-defined; however, they cause a marked increase in the time for repolarization to occur. (**Ref.** 6, pp. 754–755; **Ref.** 8, pp. 866–867; **Ref.** 9, p. 366)

248. D. Amiodarone, which prolongs the refractory period, is a class III agent, whereas disopyramide is a class Ia sodium channel blocker. (**Ref.** 1, p. 171; **Ref.** 8, p. 848; **Ref.** 9, p. 339)

249. B. Disopyramide, a class Ia antiarrhythmic agent, may produce dry mouth, constipation, and other effects observed when cholinergic function is blocked. (**Ref.** 8, p. 856; **Ref.** 9, p. 347)

250. A. Tocainide is a class Ib antiarrhythmic agent that causes nausea, vomiting, and neurologic side effects including tremor and headache. Adverse effects with bretylium include hypotension, gastrointestinal upset, and parotid pain. (**Ref.** 1, pp. 178, 792; **Ref.** 6, pp. 771–772, 776; **Ref.** 8, pp. 861, 868; **Ref.** 9, pp. 353, 365)

251. D. The class I antiarrhythmic agent associated with the production of ANA is procainamide. About 25% of patients with ANA will develop a systemic lupus erythematosus (SLE)-like syndrome. The presence of ANA alone is not a reason to discontinue therapy. (**Ref.** 1, p. 174; **Ref.** 6, pp. 765–766; **Ref.** 8, p. 856; **Ref.** 9, p. 345)

252. C. Ouabain, a quick and short-acting drug, is mainly used experimentally. The half-lives are: ouabain 21 hours, digoxin 36 hours, and digitoxin 5 days. Ouabain is given intravenously to humans occasionally. (**Ref.** 1, p. 154; **Ref.** 6, pp. 734–736; **Ref.** 8, pp. 814, 827; **Ref.** 9, p. 316)

253. A. The amount of digoxin absorbed varies from 40% to 90%, which is mainly due to the bioavailability. However, due to standards imposed by the FDA since 1974, most preparations are bioequivalent, with 75% to 80% of the digoxin absorbed. With digitoxin, 100% is usually absorbed. (**Ref.** 1, p. 154; **Ref.** 6, p. 733; **Ref.** 8, p. 828; **Ref.** 9, pp. 313–314)

254. C. The binding of cardiac glycosides to membrane Na^+, K^+-ATPase inhibits this transport enzyme. This leads to an increase in intracellular Na^{++} and a decrease in intracellular K^+ ions. Increased intracellular Na^+ stimulates $Ca^{++}-Na^+$ exchange, resulting in increased Ca^{++} within the cell. (**Ref.** 1, p. 154; **Ref.** 6, p. 719; **Ref.** 8, p. 817; **Ref.** 9, p. 310)

255. D. Both drugs increase cardiac stroke output in the failing heart. However, conflicting reports exist for the normal heart. They most likely reduce stroke output in the normal heart by limiting full relaxation during diastole, reducing the amount of blood available for expulsion during systole. (**Ref.** 3, pp. 419 420; **Ref.** 6, pp. 729–730; **Ref.** 8, pp. 825–826; **Ref.** 9, p. 312)

256. C. Both drugs increase contractile force in the normal as well as the failing heart. However, the effect is greater in the failing heart. (**Ref.** 1, p. 155; **Ref.** 3, pp. 419–420; **Ref.** 6, p. 718; **Ref.** 9, p. 312)

257. A. The doses of niacin are larger for its lowering action on triglycerides and cholesterol than is necessary for its vitamin action. These larger doses cause intense cutaneous vasodilation. This effect decreases after several weeks. (**Ref.** 1, p. 425; **Ref.** 6, pp. 834, 836; **Ref.** 8, p. 1536; **Ref.** 9, pp. 242–243)

258. A. With niacin, gastric distress frequently occurs and it is contraindicated in patients with history of peptic ulcers. Other adverse effects are decreased glucose tolerance, glycosuria, jaundice, increased plasma transaminase, and elevated plasma uric acid levels. (**Ref.** 1, p. 425; **Ref.** 6, p. 834; **Ref.** 8, p. 893; **Ref.** 9, p. 243)

259. A. The use of clofibrate and related substances leads to gallbladder problems. (**Ref.** 8, p. 889; **Ref.** 9, p. 245)

260. B. Propranolol increases and phenytoin decreases the ERP of the A – V node. In atrial flutter, atrial fibrillation, and supraventricular tachycardia, propranolol — by this action — protects the ventricles from some of the excessive stimuli, slowing the ventricular rate. (**Ref.** 6, pp. 770, 773 – 774; **Ref.** 8, pp. 865 – 866; **Ref.** 9, p. 361)

261. C. Both drugs can abolish the ventricular arrhythmias caused by digitalis toxicity; however, phenytoin and lidocaine have fewer and less dangerous adverse effects than propranolol. (**Ref.** 6, pp. 774 – 775; **Ref.** 8, p. 835; **Ref.** 9, p. 350)

262. B. Glucagon is the drug of choice in treatment of toxic effects of propranolol. Since propranolol is a competitive blocker, large doses of epinephrine or similar drug may be given in an emergency, even though this may be hazardous. (**Ref.** 8, p. 1489; **Ref.** 9, p. 363)

263. A. α_1-Acid glycoprotein in the plasma, which binds lidocaine, increases after myocardial infarction. This results in increased levels of lidocaine, but the free active levels do not increase proportionately. (**Ref.** 3, p. 442; **Ref.** 6, p. 769; **Ref.** 8, p. 851)

264. A. When used as a local anesthetic, lidocaine often contains a vasoconstrictor. Preparations for control of arrhythmias by intravenous injection should never contain adrenergic amines. (**Ref.** 6, p. 769; **Ref.** 8, p. 860)

265. C. The cardiac action of both drugs involves K^+ ions. Their actions are potentiated by hyperkalemia and are reduced by hypokalemia. (**Ref.** 1, p. 779; **Ref.** 6, pp. 762, 769; **Ref.** 8, pp. 857 – 858)

266. B. Both drugs are absorbed from the intestinal tract when administered orally; however, most of the lidocaine is metabolized on the first pass through the liver. (**Ref.** 6, pp. 759 – 761; **Ref.** 8, pp. 852, 859; **Ref.** 9, pp. 342, 348)

267. B. Quinidine prolongs the P wave, the QRS complex, and the T wave in the usual dose and to a greater extent in larger doses. Digoxin does not widen the QRS complex, it shortens the Q-T interval, and flattens or inverts the T wave; with full doses, the P-R interval is lengthened. (**Ref.** 1, p. 172; **Ref.** 3, p. 438; **Ref.** 6, pp. 722, 729, 759; **Ref.** 8, p. 851; **Ref.** 9, p. 342)

268. A. The digitalis glycosides reduce end-diastolic volume and increase the force and speed of cardiac contraction. In congestive failure, these two actions are responsible for increased cardiac output. Circulation is improved, venous pressure is reduced, tissue hypoxia is eliminated, edematous fluid is absorbed, and diuresis occurs. (**Ref.** 1, p. 153; **Ref.** 3, p. 420; **Ref.** 8, p. 825; **Ref.** 9, p. 309)

269. A. All three agents (verapamil, nifedipine, diltiazem) increase blood flow and decrease vascular resistance. Nifedipine has the greatest vasodilator action which is potentiated when used with β-blockers. (**Ref.** 8, p. 777; **Ref.** 9, p. 303)

270. E. A major side effect of calcium channel blockers is due to vasodilation, which can cause the effects listed. (**Ref.** 8, pp. 778–779; **Ref.** 9, p. 305)

271. E. Because minoxidil has little effect on the capacitance vessels its arterial vasodilation results in reflex sympathetic activation and a threefold increase in cardiac output. An interesting side effect has been increased hair growth. (**Ref.** 8, pp. 801–802; **Ref.** 9, pp. 278–279)

272. C. Inhibitors of platelet aggregation are not useful for acute management. β-Adrenergic antagonists, calcium channel blockers, and organic nitrates, not nitrites, are considered primary agents. (**Ref.** 6, p. 806; **Ref.** 8, p. 764; **Ref.** 9, p. 322)

273. E. All of the routes are employed, including transmucosal. (**Ref.** 6, pp. 810–812; **Ref.** 8, pp. 769–779; **Ref.** 9, pp. 328–329)

274. D. The use of calcium channel blockers for Prinzmetal's angina has demonstrated efficacy even though there is some disagreement over the most effective compound in the group. (**Ref.** 8, p. 779; **Ref.** 9, p. 303)

275. C. There is debate about the effectiveness of dipyridamole in angina because of its effect on various size vessels, its use for prophylaxis, and because of the feeling that it has primarily a placebo effect. (**Ref.** 1, p. 414; **Ref.** 8, p. 781; **Ref.** 9, p. 329)

276. D. The use of vasodilators usually results in the development of tolerance but their use for acute increase in cardiac output due to reduction of the load on the heart is an important aspect of their action. (**Ref.** 1, p. 161; **Ref.** 8, pp. 772, 830; **Ref.** 9, p. 319)

277. E. All of these effects can occur in addition to the simulation of almost any arrhythmia. (**Ref.** 8, p. 824)

278. C. Cardiac glycosides possess sugar molecules at position 3 which influence solubility but the basic activity resides in the genin or aglycone. A lactone group is necessary at position 17. (**Ref.** 1, pp. 153–154; **Ref.** 6, p. 717; **Ref.** 8, pp. 814–815; **Ref.** 9, p. 310)

5 Drugs Affecting Metabolic and Endocrine Functions

Hormones

DIRECTIONS (Questions 279–304): Each of the questions or incomplete statements below is followed by five suggested answers or completions. Select the **one** that is best in each case.

279. Androgens will do all of the following EXCEPT
    A. stimulate erythropoietin production
    B. provide specific androgenic effects without anabolic action
    C. provide palliative relief of advanced inoperable cancer of the breast in postmenopausal patients
    D. increase muscle mass and body weight in hypogonadism
    E. treat mild anemia

280. All the following statements about progesterone are true EXCEPT
    A. it causes a secretory endometrium following estrogen priming
    B. it binds to a specific cytosolic receptor
    C. administration leads to a decrease in body temperature
    D. it is too rapidly absorbed from oily solutions to be of optimal benefit
    E. it is secreted mainly in the second half of the menstrual cycle

281. Estrogenic activity
- **A.** is exhibited by compounds formed exclusively in the gonads, placenta, and adrenal cortices
- **B.** is evidenced by compounds with steroidal structure only
- **C.** is found in the urine of pregnant humans, pregnant mares, and stallions
- **D.** of the three main human estrogens is highest in estriol
- **E.** is inhibited by cyclic AMP

282. All of the following are adverse effects of oral contraceptives EXCEPT
- **A.** an increased incidence of cardiovascular disease with combined products
- **B.** breast engorgement and discomfort
- **C.** hypertension
- **D.** CNS stimulation and increased endurance
- **E.** thrombophlebitis is more probable with high-dose estrogen

283. All of the following statements regarding insulin/diabetes are true EXCEPT
- **A.** hypophysectomy ameliorates diabetes mellitus
- **B.** glucose administered intravenously brings about greater secretion of insulin than when it is given orally
- **C.** in the human, the normal pancreas produces from 30 to 50 units of insulin daily
- **D.** polydipsia, polyuria, and polyphagia are among obvious clinical symptoms of diabetes
- **E.** in healthy individuals the liver and the kidneys are the main sites of biodegradation of insulin

284. Regarding sulfonylurea antidiabetic drugs, all of the following statements are true EXCEPT
    A. drug sensitivity involves from 1% to 5% of patients, and cross-sensitivity among these drugs may be present
    B. with these drugs, patients who partake of alcoholic beverages may experience a disulfiram-type of reaction
    C. hypoglycemic reactions are more common among mild diabetics and may recur several days later even though the drug has been discontinued
    D. serious toxicity such as hematopoietic and hepatic effects appear to occur only rarely
    E. when administered orally absorption is quite similar for these drugs; their onset of action is about the same

285. Regarding isophane (NPH) insulin all of the following statements are true EXCEPT
    A. it is considered a type of insulin with intermediate action
    B. it has a rapid intense action that starts in about 2 hours and reaches a peak of activity in 8 to 10 hours
    C. after 10 hours it slowly has less effect, so that at 24 hours it has very little, if any, effect
    D. when isophane is administered with regular insulin, it converts it to protamine insulin because of the excess protamine present
    E. it is used in treating all diabetic states except for the initial management of diabetic ketoacidosis or diabetic emergencies

286. The mineralocorticoid activity of some of the anti-inflammatory steroids would be most likely to induce
    A. peptic ulcer
    B. hypokalemic alkalosis
    C. psychoses
    D. buffalo hump
    E. abdominal striae

287. Mestranol exerts its contraceptive action primarily by
   A. inhibiting follicle-stimulating hormone (FSH) secretion
   B. inhibiting luteinizing hormone (LH) secretion
   C. stimulating FSH secretion
   D. stimulating LH secretion
   E. inhibiting transportation of spermatozoa to the ovum

288. Chronic treatment with large doses of prednisolone may result in all of the following EXCEPT
   A. reduction of endogenous secretion of adrenocorticotropic hormone (ACTH)
   B. increased susceptibility to infections, including tuberculosis
   C. hyperglycemia and glycosuria
   D. fluid and electrolyte disturbances
   E. increased bone density

289. Corticosteroids are usually indicated in all of the following conditions EXCEPT
   A. herpes simplex of the eye
   B. status asthmaticus
   C. nephrotic syndrome
   D. collagen diseases
   E. chronic adrenal insufficiency

290. Regarding drugs affecting fertility, all of the following statements are true EXCEPT
   A. clomiphene promotes fertility in anovulatory women
   B. in combination oral contraceptives, the progestin is added primarily to stimulate the secretion of LH
   C. ethinyl estradiol possesses high oral estrogenic potency
   D. combination oral contraceptives containing high doses of estrogens can alter glucose tolerance
   E. estrogen promotes closure of the epiphyses of long bones

291. The physiologic and pharmacologic actions of estrogens include all of the following EXCEPT
    A. they cause growth and development of the vagina, uterus, and fallopian tubes
    B. they promote ductile growth of the breast
    C. the increase of estrogenic activity at the end of the menstrual cycle induces menstruation
    D. estrogens can promote salt and water retention
    E. regional pigmentation of the areola and nipples is induced by estrogens

292. An inadequate iodine intake causes
    A. decreased secretion of thyrotropin
    B. reduction in size of the thyroid gland
    C. decreased vascularity of the thyroid gland
    D. hypoplasia and atrophy of the thyroid
    E. a reduction in the ratio of thryoxine to triiodothyronine in the thyroid gland

293. All of the following facts about prolactin are true EXCEPT
    A. prolactin does not currently have a defined therapeutic use
    B. bromocriptine will inhibit prolactin secretion
    C. hyperprolactinemia may result in amenorrhea or glactorrhea
    D. there are specific receptors for prolactin in numerous tissues other than mammary gland
    E. prolactin is an antagonist of growth hormone

294. Corticotropin releasing factor (CRH)
    A. releases thyroxine from the thyroid gland
    B. releases ACTH from the pituitary
    C. releases glucocorticoids from the adrenal gland
    D. is a potentiator of hydrocortisone at tissue sites
    E. releases somatostatin

295. All of the following statements are true EXCEPT
   A. oxytocin possesses antidiuretic hormone (ADH) activity
   B. the activity of oxytocin on the uterus is increased by estrogen
   C. ADH but not oxytocin is released in response to osmolality changes
   D. oxytocin induces a contractile response of myoepithelial cells in mammary gland
   E. receptors for oxytocin in uterine smooth muscle increase during pregnancy

296. Thyroid hormones
   A. inhibit growth
   B. decrease metabolism
   C. are not considered calorigenic
   D. inhibit thyroid-stimulating hormone (TSH) release
   E. tend to decrease cardiac output

297. Hypothyroidism is preferentially treated with
   A. synthetic T_4
   B. synthetic T_3
   C. desiccated thyroid (T_3 and T_4)
   D. subcutaneous T_4
   E. intravenous T_3

298. Administration of therapeutically effective doses of iodide
   A. stimulates iodination of thyroglobulin
   B. is slow in onset usually taking 5 to 7 days
   C. destroys the thyroid gland specifically
   D. reduces vascularity of the thyroid gland
   E. is useful for long-term management of hyperthyroidism

299. Propylthiouracil
   A. accumulates in the thyroid gland
   B. stimulates thyroid hormone formation
   C. causes the thyroid gland to shrink in size
   D. inhibits active iodine transport
   E. causes iodine to accumulate in thyroglobulin

300. All of the following statements about oral contraceptives are true EXCEPT
   A. the risk factors should be evaluated for all patients
   B. patients above 30 years of age tend to have fewer risk factors
   C. oral contraceptives frequently cause nausea, dizziness, breast discomfort, and weight gain
   D. "pill" users have an increased risk of coronary thrombosis
   E. hypertension may occur in a segment of the population using oral contraception

301. Except for specific therapy, contraindications for the use of estrogens include all of the following EXCEPT
   A. endometrial cancer
   B. breast cancer
   C. liver disease
   D. thromboembolic disorder
   E. kidney disease

302. Corticosteroids
   A. possess either mineralocorticoid or glucocorticoid activity
   B. may cause severe inflammatory responses
   C. stimulate protein synthesis
   D. cause fluid retention and edema
   E. may produce hypoglycemia

303. The primary factor that regulates the secretory activity of the parathyroid gland under physiologic conditions is the
   A. concentration of ionized calcium in the circulation
   B. blood concentration of extracellular phosphate ion
   C. concentration of circulating calcitonin in the region of the gland
   D. vitamin D concentration in parathyroid cells
   E. blood concentration of a tropic hormone secreted by the anterior pituitary

304. Referring to Figure 7, which of the following statements is INCORRECT?

    A. Ovulation occurs at about day 14 of the menstrual cycle

    B. The pituitary gonadotropic hormone peaking at site 2 is luteotropic hormone (LTH), which precipitates menses

    C. The ovarian hormone that peaks at site 3 is estrogen

    D. The anterior pituitary gonadotropin that peaks at site 1 is follicle stimulating hormone (FSH) which, in addition to stimulating follicle growth and enlargement of the ovum, increases proliferation of theca cells which produce estrogen

    E. The ovarian hormone peaking at site 4 is progesterone, which is of primary importance in the development of a secretory endometrium

---

DIRECTIONS (Questions 305–323): Each group of questions below consists of five lettered headings followed by a list of numbered words, phrases, or statements. For each numbered word, phrase, or statement, select the **one** lettered heading that is most closely associated with it. Each lettered heading may be selected once, more than once, or not at all.

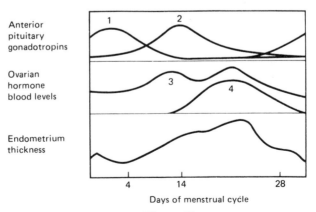

Figure 7

Questions 305–307:

    A. Aldosterone
    B. Bromocriptine
    C. Carbimazole
    D. Tamoxifen
    E. Hydrocortisone

305. Used to manage acromegaly

306. Most likely to increase susceptibility to bacterial infection

307. An antiestrogen

Questions 308 and 309:

    A. Calcium
    B. Calcitonin
    C. Sodium etidronate
    D. Vitamin D
    E. Fluoride

308. A hormone that acts to stimulate absorption of calcium and phosphate from the intestine

309. Orally effective compound for the management of Paget's disease

Questions 310 and 311:

    A. Tolbutamide
    B. Chlorpropamide
    C. Acetohexamide
    D. Tolazamide
    E. Phenformin HCl

310. Undergoes rapid biotransformation to products with considerable hypoglycemic activity

311. A derivative of sulfonylurea with a biologic half-life of approximately 35 hours

Questions 312–314:

    A. Calcitonin
    B. Propranolol
    C. Lugol's solution (strong iodine solution, USP)
    D. Radioactive iodine
    E. Methimazole

312. Its usefulness in treatment of hyperthyroidism is the result of inhibition of thyroid peroxidase and blockade of thyroid peroxidase-catalyzed iodination of thyroglobulin

313. Valuable in controlling symptoms of thyrotoxicosis while awaiting the response to radioiodine and may be very useful in treating patients experiencing thyroid storm

314. Large doses paradoxically cause rapid inhibition of thyroid hormone secretion in euthyroid individuals, experimental animals, and hyperthyroid patients—an action that may be responsible for its usefulness in the treatment of Graves' disease

Questions 315–319:

    A. Aldosterone
    B. Prednisone
    C. Dexamethasone
    D. Fluonisolide
    E. Metapyrone

315. Inhibits cytochrome P_{450} enzymes

316. Prototype mineralocorticoid

317. Reduced in the liver to a compound with approximately the same activity

318. A steroid given by inhalation

319. A glucocorticoid used orally which has a long duration of action relative to other agents

Questions 320–323:

    A. Tolbutamide
    B. Glipizide
    C. NPH insulin
    D. Glucagon
    E. Ultralente insulin

320. A second-generation sulfonylurea

321. May be used for severe hypoglycemia

322. This compound has a long (24 hours) duration of action coupled with a very slow (6 hours) onset of action

323. A compound that is reported to increase cardiovascular mortality when compared with insulin

---

DIRECTIONS (Questions 324–329): Each set of lettered headings below is followed by a list of numbered words or phrases. For each numbered word or phrase select

    A if the item is associated with **A** only
    B if the item is associated with **B** only
    C if the item is associated with both **A** and **B**
    D if the item is associated with neither **A** nor **B**

Questions 324–327:

    A. Androgen
    B. Estrogen
    C. Both
    D. Neither

324. Exerts an inhibitory action on cephalic hair growth in females

325. Augments fusion of the epiphyses

326. Synthesized by the ovary

327. Increases libido in normal men

Questions 328 and 329:

    A. Single dose of 1 mg of l-triiodothyronine
    B. Single dose of 4 mg of l-thyroxine
    C. Both
    D. Neither

328. Metabolic response occurs in 4 to 6 hours

329. The effect outlasts the presence of detectable elevated amounts of hormone in the blood

Drugs Affecting Blood and Blood-Forming Organs

DIRECTIONS (Questions 330–334): Each of the questions or incomplete statements below is followed by five suggested answers or completions. Select the **one** that is best in each case.

330. When iron is to be given parenterally
    A. the intramuscular route is the most desirable avenue of administration
    B. the most serious side effects that are likely to be encountered when given intravenously are generalized lymphadenopathy and arthralgias
    C. the preparation most widely used in the United States is iron dextran injection
    D. the intramuscular route affords a highly desirable repository form of iron since 10% to 50% of such a dose may become fixed locally in the muscle for many months
    E. one may be certain that iron so administered will produce a pharmacologic response more rapidly than if it is given orally

331. The major component of body iron is in
   A. the protein hemoglobin
   B. the globulin transferrin
   C. myoglobin
   D. ferritin, the storage form of iron in tissues
   E. cytochrome enzymes

332. All of the following statements concerning vitamin B_{12} are true EXCEPT
   A. it is not inherently present in higher plants
   B. man depends on exogenous sources of supply
   C. it is preferentially stored in parenchymal cells of the liver, and the supply of vitamin B_{12} available for tissues is directly related to the size of the hepatic storage pool
   D. intracellular vitamin B_{12} is maintained as two active coenzymes, methylcobalamin and deoxyadenosyl-cobalamin
   E. in humans, the daily nutritional requirement is provided by synthesis in the gastrointestinal tract

333. Which of the following statements concerning erythropoietin is **NOT** true?
   A. Erythropoietin is effective in treating anemia of chronic renal failure
   B. The action of erythropoietin is receptor mediated
   C. There is a high incidence of allergic reactions when erythropoietin is administered
   D. There is a constant level of erythropoietin in plasma
   E. Cancer chemotherapy-induced anemia can be treated with erythropoietin

334. In hematopoiesis
   A. growth factors are very specific for cell type
   B. growth factors have limited action at one part of the proliferation process
   C. growth factors exert delicate control of both hemato-poiesis and lymphopoiesis
   D. the process of proliferation of colony-forming units is under the exclusive control of IL-3
   E. at steady state the level of blood cells produced is less than 200 million/day

DIRECTIONS (Questions 335–340): Each group of questions below consists of five lettered headings followed by a list of numbered words, phrases, or statements. For each numbered word, phrase, or statement, select the **one** lettered heading that is most closely associated with it. Each lettered heading may be selected once, more than once, or not at all.

Questions 335–337:

    A. Vitamin B_{12}
    B. Folic acid
    C. Ferrous sulfate
    D. Heparin
    E. Tissue plasminogen activator (t-PA)

335. A thrombolytic agent

336. A characteristic of this compound is the electronegative charge

337. In a deficiency state, only the megaloblastic anemia but not the neurologic symptoms are corrected by this agent

Questions 338–340:

    A. Granulocyte/macrophage-colony stimulating factor (GM-CSF)
    B. Heparin
    C. Aspirin
    D. G-CSF
    E. Streptokinase

338. Administration leads to an increase in circulating neutrophils, monocytes, and eosinophils

339. Permanent inhibitor of thromboxane A_2 (TXA_2) production

340. Routinely used to inhibit clot formation in tubing and cannulae

---

DIRECTIONS (Questions 341–347): For each of the questions or incomplete statements below, **one** or **more** of the answers or completions given is correct. Select

    A if only 1, 2, and 3 are correct
    B if only 1 and 3 are correct
    C if only 2 and 4 are correct
    D if only 4 is correct
    E if all are correct

---

341. Regarding the therapeutic use of iron
    1. oral ferrous sulfate is the treatment of choice for iron deficiency
    2. oral iron salts differ very little in their bioavailability
    3. because absorption of iron is crucially dependent on the dose administered, the largest dose tolerated without side effects should be given
    4. medicinal iron preparations are relatively nontoxic for children

342. Regarding anticoagulant properties of acetylsalicylic acid
    1. low-dose (0.3 g) aspirin causes marked increases in bleeding time
    2. aspirin has been shown to be highly effective in secondary prevention of myocardial infarction
    3. its anticoagulant effect is related to cyclooxygenase inhibition
    4. anticoagulant effects are decreased in vitamin K deficiency

	Directions Summarized			
A	B	C	D	E
1,2,3	1,3	2,4	4	All are
only	only	only	only	correct

343. Photophobia, lacrimation, stomatitis, cheilosis, and keratitis characterize a deficiency of
    1. ascorbic acid
    2. vitamin B_2
    3. vitamin B_6
    4. riboflavin

344. Isotretinoin, or 13-*cis*-retinoic acid, is a vitamin A derivative which
    1. temporarily suppresses activity of sebaceous glands
    2. is highly effective in clearing severe nodulocystic acne
    3. is administered orally, but should be restricted to cases that do not respond to conventional therapy
    4. has caused major fetal abnormalities and spontaneous abortion

345. The mechanism of action of the anticoagulant effect of coumarin derivatives involves
    1. a reduction in levels of factors VII, IX, and X
    2. an action taking place in the bloodstream
    3. an interference with the action of vitamin K
    4. mainly an action to block the release of preformed prothrombin by the liver

346. Folic acid
    1. is a designation for pteroylglutamic acid
    2. occurs in nature as folate, primarily as a conjugate with glutamic acid
    3. has a daily requirement in normal human adults of less than 100 μg
    4. is active in the body as pteroylglutamic acid

347. Iron deficiency
    1. may be the cause of anemia following hookworm infestation
    2. may result from nutritional deficiency
    3. results from chronic blood loss
    4. occurs more often in women

Vitamins

DIRECTIONS (Questions 348–356): Each of the questions or incomplete statements below is followed by five suggested answers or completions. Select the **one** that is best in each case.

348. Regarding vitamins, all of the following statements are true EXCEPT
    A. vitamin deficiency is usually not specific for one vitamin but is a nutritional deficiency in which several vitamins are lacking
    B. vitamin supplementation is not generally necessary except for defined special risk groups, ie, pregnancy, elderly
    C. fat-soluble vitamins include A, C, D, E, and K
    D. the term vitamin refers to chemical substances that are necessary in small amounts for growth, metabolism, and development
    E. water-soluble vitamins are rapidly metabolized and excreted in the urine

349. All of the following facts about vitamin A are true EXCEPT
   A. it improves vision in dim light
   B. it is useful in the prophylaxis of certain malignancies
   C. different forms of the molecule mediate different functions
   D. epithelial cell differentiation is inhibited by vitamin A
   E. large tissue reserves are present and deficiency is not noted until deprivation is of long-standing duration

350. Vitamin C
   A. megadoses are useful in preventing the common cold
   B. prevents kidney stones
   C. is necessary for collagen synthesis
   D. is low in fresh fruits
   E. is another name for folic acid

351. All of the following are members of the vitamin B complex EXCEPT
   A. retinoic acid
   B. riboflavin
   C. thiamine
   D. cyanocobalamin
   E. pyridoxine

352. All of the following statements about vitamin D are correct EXCEPT
   A. the major role of vitamin D is to provide a positive influence on calcium ion
   B. vitamin D_3 is formed in the skin
   C. the major source of vitamin D in humans is skin irradiation by sunlight
   D. the principal result of vitamin D deficiency is scurvy
   E. hypervitaminosis D is characterized by hypercalcemia

353. All of the following statements about absorption of vitamins are correct EXCEPT
    A. bile is necessary for absorption of vitamin D
    B. vitamin E enters the blood in chylomicrons
    C. retinol absorption occurs by a carrier-mediated process
    D. ascorbic is readily and completely absorbed from the gastrointestinal (GI) tract
    E. compounds with vitamin K activity require bile for absorption

354. Vitamin A toxicity may cause
    A. teratogenicity
    B. renal stones
    C. impairment of pain, touch, and temperature sensation
    D. flushing and GI disturbances
    E. bleeding

355. Vitamin E is
    A. riboflavin
    B. isotriniton
    C. carotene
    D. biotin
    E. α-tocopherol

356. Vitamin D (cholecalciferol)
    A. is obtained from the diet
    B. is converted to the hormone 7-dehydrocholesterol
    C. is also known as 25-hydroxy D_3, which is devoid of biologic activity
    D. circulates freely in blood
    E. is eventually converted to 1,25-dihydroxy D_3, the most active form of the vitamin

DIRECTIONS (Questions 357–359): The set of lettered headings below is followed by a list of numbered words or phrases. For each numbered word or phrase select

    A if the item is associated with **A** only
    B if the item is associated with **B** only
    C if the item is associated with both **A** and **B**
    D if the item is associated with neither **A** nor **B**

    A. Thiamine
    B. Nicotinic acid
    C. Both
    D. Neither

357. Member of the B-complex group of vitamins

358. A deficiency in intake can lead to scurvy, a disease characterized by abnormalities in the connective tissue

359. Its biologic metabolites serve a vital role as coenzymes for a variety of proteins that catalyze oxidation–reduction reactions essential for tissue respiration

DIRECTIONS (Questions 360–363): For each of the questions or incomplete statements below, **one** or **more** of the answers or completions given is correct. Select

    A if only 1, 2, and 3 are correct
    B if only 1 and 3 are correct
    C if only 2 and 4 are correct
    D if only 4 is correct
    E if all are correct

360. Regarding vitamins
    1. pyridoxine alters the metabolism of levodopa, reducing its effectiveness
    2. vitamin C deficiency leads to multiple minute hemorrhages
    3. thiamine deficiency results in the disease beriberi
    4. vitamin K enhances the anticoagulant property of coumarins

361. Swollen and tender joints, gingival bleeding, increased tooth mobility, and impaired healing of small cuts and bruises are symptoms often associated with
1. niacin deficiency
2. ascorbic acid deficiency
3. hypervitaminosis E
4. scurvy

362. The symptoms of glossitis with a swollen fiery red tongue, enteritis, diarrhea, and CNS depression are associated with
1. scurvy
2. nicotinic acid deficiency
3. hypovitaminosis A
4. niacin deficiency

363. Ecchymoses, epistaxis, hematuria, and gastrointestinal bleeding best characterize a deficiency of
1. vitamin C
2. vitamin D
3. vitamin E
4. vitamin K

Explanatory Answers

279. B. All anabolic hormones currently known have androgenic effects. (**Ref.** 1, p. 512; **Ref.** 3, p. 596; **Ref.** 6, pp. 1452–1454; **Ref.** 8, pp. 1424–1426)

280. C. Progesterone is thermogenic. (**Ref.** 1, p. 499; **Ref.** 6, pp. 1426–1427; **Ref.** 8, p. 1399)

281. C. The largest source of natural estrogens is in the urine of a stallion. Liver, skeletal muscle, and other tissues also form estrogens. (**Ref.** 6, pp. 1412–1413; **Ref.** 8, p. 1385)

282. D. Oral contraceptives may cause depression and a sense of fatigue. This effect may be less in new low-dose preparations. (**Ref.** 1, p. 505; **Ref.** 6, pp. 1434–1435; **Ref.** 8, p. 1408)

283. B. When glucose is given orally, greater amounts of insulin are secreted apparently because of liberation of gastrin, secretin, pancreozymin, and "gut" glucagon. (**Ref.** 6, pp. 1490, 1493; **Ref.** 8, p. 1466, **Ref.** 9, p. 939)

284. E. Their durations of action are: acetohexamide 12–24 hours, tolbutamide 6–12 hours, chlorpropamide up to 60 hours, and tolazamide 10–14 hours. (**Ref.** 1, p. 525; **Ref.** 6, pp. 1505–1507)

285. D. In NPH insulin, there is no excess protamine; each 100 units of regular insulin contains 0.5 mg protamine. This is just enough protamine to bind the regular insulin. (**Ref.** 1, p. 522; **Ref.** 6, pp. 1501–1502)

286. B. Mineralocorticoids favor the retention of sodium and water and excretion of potassium, leading to hypokalemic alkalosis and edema. (**Ref.** 1, p. 488; **Ref.** 6, pp. 1468, 1478–1479; **Ref.** 8, p. 1439)

287. A. The predominant effect of the estrogen mestranol is to inhibit the secretion of FSH by a negative feedback mechanism. (**Ref.** 6, p. 1431; **Ref.** 8, p. 1405; **Ref.** 9, p. 882)

288. E. Osteoporosis, a frequent serious complication of prolonged corticosteroid therapy in patients of all ages, is an indication for withdrawal of therapy. (**Ref.** 6, p. 1479; **Ref.** 8, p. 1452; **Ref.** 9, p. 866)

289. A. Corticosteroids are contraindicated in herpes simplex (dendritic keratitis) of the eye because progression of the disease and irreversible clouding of the cornea may occur. (**Ref.** 1, p. 486; **Ref.** 6, pp. 1481 – 1483; **Ref.** 8, p. 1456)

290. B. Progestin suppresses ovulation by inhibition of LH through interference with hypothalamic – pituitary mechanisms. (**Ref.** 3, p. 592; **Ref.** 8, p. 1405)

291. C. A decline in estrogenic activity at the end of the menstrual cycle actually brings about menstruation. (**Ref.** 6, p. 1414; **Ref.** 8, p. 1386)

292. E. In the absence of adequate amounts of iodine, thyroid hormone secretion increases, the gland increases in size and vascularity, thyrotropin secretion is inhibited, and the ratio of thyroxine to triiodothyronine is reduced. (**Ref.** 6, p. 1395; **Ref.** 8, p. 1367)

293. E. The physiologic effects of prolactin, a polypeptide which has actions similar to growth hormone, are far reaching. (**Ref.** 8, pp. 1344 – 1346; **Ref.** 9, pp. 848 – 849)

294. B. CRH is a hypothalamic polypeptide which causes the release of ACTH, which then acts on the adrenal gland. (**Ref.** 8, p. 1356; **Ref.** 9, p. 851)

295. C. Oxytocin has very close structural similarity to ADH as well as some overlap in function and both polypeptides are released in response to osmotic alterations. (**Ref.** 8, pp. 835 – 836; **Ref.** 9, pp. 853 – 854)

296. D. With the exception of TSH release, which is inhibited (negative feedback), the calorigenic hormones, T_4 and/or T_3, stimulate growth and metabolism. Cardiac output is increased when thyroid levels are elevated. (**Ref.** 1, pp. 469–470; **Ref.** 3, p. 561; **Ref.** 8, pp. 1367, 1369; **Ref.** 9, p. 914)

297. A. Thyroid hormones are orally effective and are normally administered by mouth except in a myxedema coma, where intravenous T_3 is used. T_4 is the preferred agent. (**Ref.** 1, p. 471; **Ref.** 3, p. 563; **Ref.** 8, p. 1371; **Ref.** 9, pp. 915–917)

298. D. Iodide administration can be used to reduce vascularity and cause the thyroid gland to become firm prior to surgery. Its onset occurs within 24 hours but it cannot suppress hyperthyroidism indefinitely. (**Ref.** 1, p. 472; **Ref.** 3, p. 564; **Ref.** 8, pp. 1377–1378; **Ref.** 9, p. 922)

299. A. Antithyroid drugs like propylthiouracil and methimazole accumulate in the gland and inhibit iodination of thyroglobulin. These agents do not block iodine transport. The gland may undergo hypertrophy. (**Ref.** 1, pp. 471–472; **Ref.** 3, pp. 564–565; **Ref.** 8, pp. 1374–1375; **Ref.** 9, pp. 920–921)

300. B. The use of oral contraceptives is associated with a number of serious adverse effects on the cardiovascular system along with some troublesome effects such as nausea, headache, and some symptoms resembling early pregnancy. Overall, in patients below the age of 30 who do not have risk factors, they are relatively safe. (**Ref.** 1, pp. 504–505; **Ref.** 8, pp. 1406–1409)

301. E. It is recognized that estrogens should not be used in cancer or suspected cancer even though some forms of cancer respond favorably to high doses of estrogen. Thromboembolism or liver disease are also contraindications but there is no evidence they are contraindicated in kidney disease. (**Ref.** 1, p. 498; **Ref.** 3, p. 590; **Ref.** 9, p. 890)

302. D. Corticosteroids have anti-inflammatory activity and far-reaching metabolic effects resulting in decreased protein synthesis (negative nitrogen balance) and hyperglycemia. There is an arbitrary distinction between mineralocorticoids and glucocorticoids, but this is only relative. (**Ref.** 8, pp. 1436–1437; **Ref.** 9, p. 859)

303. A. Although it is not clear whether the extracellular calcium or the ionized calcium in the parathyroid cells is the actual "trigger" for release of hormone, the output of parathyroid hormone is apparently regulated by the level of serum calcium acting through a feedback mechanism. (**Ref.** 3, p. 567; **Ref.** 6, p. 1526; **Ref.** 8, p. 1504)

304. B. Although prolactin, once called luteotropin, may play a role in the menstrual cycle, its precise function in this respect is not presently known; the surge of luteinizing hormone (LH) is of primary importance in causing rupture of the follicle. (**Ref.** 1, pp. 149, 493; **Ref.** 3, pp. 584–586; **Ref.** 6, pp. 1373, 1414, 1416, 1426; **Ref.** 8, pp. 1344, 1348, 1387)

305. B. Tumors of the pituitary that secrete excessive growth hormone can be inhibited by dopaminergic agonists like bromocriptine. (**Ref.** 6, p. 1374; **Ref.** 8, p. 1346)

306. E. Glucocorticoids impair defense mechanisms against infections and increase the susceptibility to bacterial pathogens and fungal pathogens. (**Ref.** 3, p. 551; **Ref.** 6, p. 1478; **Ref.** 8, p. 1448; **Ref.** 9, p. 865)

307. D. Tamoxifen and clomiphene are two antiestrogens being utilized to treat infertility. (**Ref.** 1, p. 506; **Ref.** 6, pp. 1423–1424; **Ref.** 8, pp. 1395–1396; **Ref.** 9, pp. 877, 884)

308. D. Vitamin D is now recognized as a hormone. It increases absorption of calcium and phosphate from the gut, decreases their excretion, and enhances bone resorption. Parathyroid hormone increases intestinal absorption indirectly through calcitriol and directly through an unknown mechanism. (**Ref.** 1, pp. 532–534; **Ref.** 3, pp. 567–568; **Ref.** 6, pp. 1517, 1527, 1531; **Ref.** 8, pp. 1506, 1510, 1512)

309. C. Sodium etidronate has an advantage over calcitonin in that it is inexpensive, orally effective, and nonantigenic. (**Ref.** 6, p. 1531; **Ref.** 8, p. 1509)

310. C. The principal metabolite is hydroxyhexamide which has a metabolic half-life that is considerably longer than the biologic half-life of the sulfonylurea drugs. (**Ref.** 1, p. 526; **Ref.** 6, p. 1505; **Ref.** 8, p. 1486; **Ref.** 9, pp. 948–949)

311. B. The kidneys excrete chlorpropamide slowly, eliminating 80% to 90% of a single oral dose within 4 days. Usually 5 days of drug administration is required to reach a steady state, and up to 20 days are required for complete elimination if drug administration is stopped. (**Ref.** 1, pp. 525–526; **Ref.** 6, p. 1505; **Ref.** 8, p. 1486; **Ref.** 9, p. 950)

312. E. The tioamides compete with tyrosine residues of thyroglobulin for active iodine and also inactive thyroid peroxidase. (**Ref.** 1, p. 472; **Ref.** 8, p. 1374; **Ref.** 9, p. 920)

313. B. The increased heart rate, palpitation, anxiety, tension, tremor, and stare associated with hyperthyroidism are rapidly controlled by oral administration of propranolol. (**Ref.** 3, p. 566; **Ref.** 6, p. 1404; **Ref.** 8, p. 1376; **Ref.** 9, p. 923)

314. C. Iodide is the first substance known to have been used successfully in treatment of thyroid disorders, an effect that remains paradoxical since increased iodide intake would be expected to result in an increase rather than a decrease in thyroid hormone synthesis. (**Ref.** 1, p. 472; **Ref.** 6, pp. 1405–1406; **Ref.** 8, p. 1377)

315. E. Metapyrone is an inhibitor of glucocorticoid synthesis leading to increased ACTH production. It can be used to test pituitary function and to suppress excess glucocorticoid production in specific situations. (**Ref.** 1, p. 490; **Ref.** 8, p. 1458; **Ref.** 9, p. 870)

316. A. Aldosterone is the most potent glucocorticoid synthesized by the adrenal cortex that influences salt and water balance. (**Ref.** 1, p. 487; **Ref.** 3, p. 555; **Ref.** 8, pp. 1437, 1440; **Ref.** 9, p. 859)

317. B. Prednisolone is prednisone with the 11-keto group reduced to a hydroxyl group. These compounds are used interchangeably. (**Ref.** 8, p. 1447; **Ref.** 9, p. 963)

318. D. Fluonisolide is a steroid given by inhalation for management of bronchial asthma. The approach allows for less systemic effect when using glucocorticoids for anti-inflammatory treatment of asthma. (**Ref.** 8, p. 1456; **Ref.** 9, pp. 610–611)

319. C. Dexamethasone and betamethasone are orally effective glucocorticoids with a biologic half-life of 3 to 4 days. (**Ref.** 1, p. 462; **Ref.** 8, p. 1447; **Ref.** 9, p. 864)

320. B. Glipizide is an oral hypoglycemic agent which requires the presence of pancreatic β cells for its action. It is approximately 100 times the potency of tolbutamide. (**Ref.** 1, pp. 525–527; **Ref.** 3, p. 540; **Ref.** 8, pp. 1485–1486; **Ref.** 9, pp. 947–948)

321. D. The administration of glucagon, which is synthesized in the A cells of the pancreatic islets of Langerhans, causes hyperglycemia through hepatic glycolysis. (**Ref.** 1, p. 529; **Ref.** 3, p. 534; **Ref.** 8, p. 1488)

322. E. The zinc 943 crystals of insulin, called ultralente, are similar to protamine zinc insulin in onset and duration of action. (**Ref.** 1, p. 520; **Ref.** 8, p. 1477; **Ref.** 9, p. 946)

323. A. The University Group Diabetes Program (UGDP) reported this still unresolved adverse effect of tolbutamide in the early 1970s. Today package inserts warn patients about the findings of this report. (**Ref.** 1, pp. 525–526; **Ref.** 8, p. 1486)

324. A. Androgen increases body hair, but has the potential to bring about patterns of male baldness when administered to females. (**Ref.** 6, p. 1450; **Ref.** 8, p. 1420; **Ref.** 9, p. 906)

325. C. Both androgen and estrogen bring about closure of the epiphyses. (**Ref.** 6, pp. 1414, 1450; **Ref.** 8, pp. 1386, 1416; **Ref.** 9, pp. 879, 898)

326. C. Both androgen and estrogen are synthesized, not only in the ovary, but in the testis as well. Fractionation of steroids contained in venous ovarian blood indicates that both testosterone and androstenedione, precursors of estrogens, are normal ovarian secretions. (**Ref.** 6, pp. 1414, 1443; **Ref.** 8, pp. 1387, 1416)

327. D. In normal men, androgens do not increase libido. Estrogens have a negative effect. (**Ref.** 6, p. 1452; **Ref.** 8, p. 1424)

328. A. The more rapid action of T_3 may make it useful in certain situations, such as hypothyroidism resulting from drug therapy or surgery, when a quicker action is needed. (**Ref.** 6, pp. 1393–1394, 1399, 1400; **Ref.** 8, p. 1371; **Ref.** 9, p. 917)

329. C. When T_4 is given in a dose four times greater than that of T_3, the elevation of metabolic rate produced by each is about equal and the effects of both continue after their disappearance from the blood. (**Ref.** 6, p. 1399; **Ref.** 8, p. 1372)

330. C. Although another form of iron for parenteral use is available in Europe, iron dextran is in general use in the United States at present. When specific indications for parenteral use of iron are present, the intravenous route is preferable to the intramuscular route because of the hazards of iron deposition in tissues. (**Ref.** 6, pp. 1317–1318; **Ref.** 8, p. 1292)

331. A. Hemoglobin, which contains the major part, in combination with ferritin, holds the bulk of the total body iron, leaving only trace amounts at each of the other sites. (**Ref.** 6, p. 1309; **Ref.** 8, p. 1283)

332. E. Vitamin B_{12} is synthesized in the large bowel of humans, but it is unavailable for absorption, and a daily nutritional requirement of 3 to 5 μg must be obtained from animal by-products in the diet. (**Ref.** 6, pp. 1323, 1325–1326; **Ref.** 8, pp. 1296–1297)

333. C. The growth factor erythropoietin does not result in allergic reactions. (**Ref.** 8, pp. 1279–1281)

334. C. The process of hematopoiesis and lymphopoiesis (200 billion cells/day) is delicate; it is also a complex process involving networking and action at multiple steps providing for synergistic interactions. (**Ref.** 8, p. 1279)

335. E. t-PA is a recombinant DNA technology protease which is useful in the lysing thrombi formed in myocardial infarction. (**Ref.** 8, p. 1324; **Ref.** 9, p. 384)

336. D. Heparin is a mixture of mucopolysaccharides which act intravenously as anticoagulants. The activity is inhibited by the electropositive compound protamine. (**Ref.** 8, pp. 1313, 1317; **Ref.** 9, pp. 372, 374)

337. B. Folic acid corrects the megaloblastic anemia of B_{12} deficiency; however, the neurologic symptoms may progress. (**Ref.** 8, p. 1305; **Ref.** 9, p. 1001)

338. A. Granulocyte/macrophage-colony stimulating factor will increase the proliferation of these cell lines in the bone marrow. (**Ref.** 8, p. 1282)

339. C. Aspirin inhibits cyclooxygenase in platelets which cannot synthesize protein, hence the TXA_2 production causing vasoconstriction is permanently inhibited. (**Ref.** 8, p. 1325; **Ref.** 9, p. 379)

340. B. Since heparin is effective in vitro it can be added to blood or placed in the blood to inhibit clot formation in and at sites where blood is passed through tubing or machines and/or where a cannula is in-place. (**Ref.** 8, p. 1336; **Ref.** 9, p. 373)

341. B. In most instances, oral ferrous sulfate is the preferred treatment of iron-deficiency anemia, and it is relatively inexpensive. However, iron tablets may cause serious toxicity in children. (**Ref.** 6, pp. 1314–1317; **Ref.** 8, pp. 1289–1291)

342. B. The use of low-dose aspirin to prevent myocardial infarction and stroke is controversial. However, it does decrease vascular mortality (15%). This use is based on its anticoagulant effect due to inhibition of production of thromboxane A_2. Vitamin K antagonizes this effect of aspirin. (**Ref.** 1, p. 413; **Ref.** 6, pp. 683, 1352; **Ref.** 8, pp. 653, 1329)

343. C. In addition to the listed symptoms, riboflavin, or vitamin B_2, deficiency may produce anemia, which may be related to disturbances in folic acid metabolism. The physiologically active forms of riboflavin, FMN and FAD, serve a vital role in metabolism as coenzymes for a wide variety of respiratory proteins. (**Ref.** 6, pp. 1555–1556; **Ref.** 8, pp. 1534–1535)

344. E. Isotretinoin is reputed to be the most effective treatment yet discovered for acne. However, its use should be restricted to cases where other approaches have failed. Birth defects and spontaneous abortion leads to serious cause for concern especially as young women of childbearing age are often troubled by acne. (**Ref. 6**, p. 1581; **Ref. 8**, p. 1577)

345. B. The oral anticoagulants have no effect on the clotting factors that are already formed, but rather interfere with the action of vitamin K in the synthesis of factors II, VII, IX, and X. (**Ref. 6**, p. 1345; **Ref. 8**, p. 1317)

346. A. Folic acid is pteroylglutamic acid, but it is neither the principal folate congener nor the active coenzyme for cellular metabolism. (**Ref. 1**, pp. 400–401; **Ref. 6**, pp. 1332–1333; **Ref. 8**, p. 1302)

347. E. All of the above may be causes of iron-deficiency anemia, which occurs in pre-postmenopausal women due to menstruation and pregnancy. (**Ref. 8**, p. 1287; **Ref. 9**, p. 1001)

348. C. All answers are true except that the fat-soluble vitamins are A, D, E, and K, whereas the water-soluble vitamins are the B-complex and C. (**Ref. 8**, pp. 1524, 1528, 1530, 1553; **Ref. 9**, pp. 993–995)

349. D. Vitamin A is necessary for differentiation and proliferation of epithelial cells. The lack of vitamin A leads to hyperplasia and a lack of differentiation. (**Ref. 8**, pp. 1554, 1557; **Ref. 9**, pp. 993–998)

350. C. There is no solid evidence that vitamin C (ascorbic acid) cures the common cold; however, it does cause kidney stones, is high in fresh fruits and vegetables, and is necessary for collagen synthesis. (**Ref. 8**, pp. 1548–1550; **Ref. 9**, pp. 994–995, 999)

351. A. Retinoic acid is in the A vitamin category. B_1 is thiamine, B_2 is riboflavin, B_6 is pyridoxine, and cyanocobalamin is B_{12}. (**Ref. 8**, pp. 1294, 1530, 1534, 1538, 1554; **Ref. 9**, p. 994)

352. D. The disease rickets results from a lack of vitamin D. Scurvy is due to vitamin C deficiency. (**Ref.** 8, pp. 1510, 1514; **Ref.** 9, pp. 993–994, 997–998)

353. E. There are various compounds containing vitamin K activity. Phytonadione requires bile but menadione does not; it is water soluble. (**Ref.** 8, pp. 1515, 1559, 1564–1565, 1569)

354. A. Renal stones may be caused by overdoses of vitamin C. Pyridoxine causes sensation changes. Nicotinic acid causes flushing and a deficiency of vitamin K causes bleeding. Teratogenic effects can occur with large doses of vitamin A. (**Ref.** 9, p. 998)

355. E. While there are several tocopherols, α-tocopherol is the most prevalent in animal tissues. It serves as an antioxidant. (**Ref.** 8, p. 1567; **Ref.** 9, p. 997)

356. E. Ultraviolet sunlight converts dietary 7-dehydrocholesterol to the prohormone D_3 which then is altered in the liver to 25-hydroxy D_3 and in the kidney to 1,25 dihydroxy D_3, which is bound to transport proteins in the blood. (**Ref.** 8, pp. 1511, 1515; **Ref.** 9, p. 929)

357. C. Traditionally, there are 11 members of the vitamin B complex, including thiamine and nicotinic acid, which are grouped in a single class because of their original isolation from the same sources, notably liver and yeast. (**Ref.** 6, p. 1551; **Ref.** 8, p. 1530)

358. D. Scurvy is a disease state resulting from a deficiency of vitamin C; the disease caused by nicotinic acid deficiency is pellagra. (**Ref.** 6, pp. 1557, 1567; **Ref.** 8, pp. 1537, 1549)

359. B. Nicotinic acid is converted in the body to its physiologically active forms, NAD and NADP, which function as oxidants accepting electrons and hydrogen from substrates. (**Ref.** 6, p. 1558; **Ref.** 8, p. 1536)

360. A. Vitamin K is a competitive antagonist of anticoagulant drugs such as dicoumarol and its derivatives. The excessive hypo-prothrombinemia and bleeding produced by coumarins are corrected rapidly by the administration of vitamin K. (**Ref.** 6, pp. 1350, 1553, 1561, 1569; **Ref.** 8, pp. 1532, 1539, 1549, 1566)

361. C. Vitamin C, or ascorbic acid, deficiency leads to scurvy. The chief lesions of scurvy arise in the bones and blood vessels. The primary structural changes in vitamin C deficiency result from the fact that ascorbic acid is essential for the formation and maintenance of intercellular ground substance and collagen. (**Ref.** 6, pp. 1568–1569; **Ref.** 8, pp. 1548–1549)

362. C. Niacin, or nicotinic acid, deficiency is observed in the CNS, the skin, and the digestive tract. GI symptoms are stomatitis, enteritis, and diarrhea. Niacin serves a vital role in metabolism as coenzyme for a wide variety of proteins involved in tissue respiration. (**Ref.** 6, p. 1558; **Ref.** 8, pp. 1536–1538)

363. D. Vitamin K deficiency is associated primarily with hemorrhagic manifestations. The normal physiologic function is to promote biosynthesis of prothrombin (factor II), proconvertin (factor VII), plasma thromboplastin component (factor X), and the Stuart factor. (**Ref.** 1, pp. 415–416; **Ref.** 3, p. 994; **Ref.** 6, p. 1583; **Ref.** 8, p. 1564)

6 Drugs Acting on the Central Nervous System

General Anesthetics

DIRECTIONS (Questions 364–367): Each of the questions or incomplete statements below is followed by five suggested answers or completions. Select the **one** best in each case.

364. Given the following blood:gas partition coefficients, which of the following should be associated with the agent that induces anesthesia the most rapidly?
    A. 0.15
    B. 0.47
    C. 1.4
    D. 2.4
    E. 11

365. The halogenated anesthetic methoxyflurane
    A. elevates arterial blood pressure
    B. increases myocardial contractile force
    C. reduces heart rate
    D. does not sensitize the myocardium to catecholamines
    E. increases sympathetic nervous system activity

366. The sedative-hypnotic agents, the diazepams given intravenously, are used to induce anesthesia and when compared with intravenous barbiturates
   A. give a slower onset of anesthesia
   B. yield a longer postoperative period of amnesia
   C. tend to give light anesthesia
   D. have a shorter postoperative recovery period
   E. all of the above

367. All of the following are complications and undesirable features associated with the use of intravenous barbiturates EXCEPT
   A. danger of tissue necrosis from extravascular administration
   B. respiratory depression and apnea
   C. laryngospasm
   D. circulatory depression from overdose
   E. increased salivary secretion

DIRECTIONS (Questions 368–371): Each group of questions below consist of five lettered headings followed by a list of numbered words, phrases, or statements. For each numbered word, phrase, or statement, select the **one** lettered heading that is most closely associated with it. Each lettered heading may be selected once, more than once, or not at all.

Questions 368–371:

   A. Halothane
   B. Enflurane
   C. Methoxyflurane
   D. Isoflurane
   E. Nitrous oxide

368. The most potent of the inhalation anesthetic agents

369. Seizures may occur during deep anesthesia with this agent, especially when hypocapnia is present

370. Unlike the other halogenated compounds listed above, myocardial function is well maintained during anesthesia with this agent

371. Only one of these five agents that does not decrease respiratory rate or tidal volume

---

DIRECTIONS (Questions 372–378): Each group of questions below consists of a diagram or table with three or four lettered components, followed by a list of numbered words, phrases, or statements. For each numbered word, phrase, or statement, select the **one** lettered component that is most closely associated with it. Each lettered component may be selected once, more than once, or not at all.

Questions 372–375 (Figure 8):

372. Brain, heart, and kidney

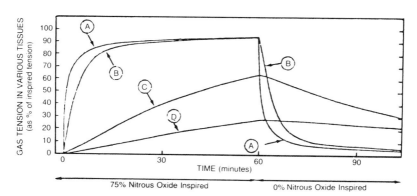

Figure 8 Tissue tensions of an anesthetic gas during uptake and elimination. (Reproduced from Smith TC, Wollman H: History and principles of anesthesiology, in Gilman AG, Goodman LS, Rall TW, Murad F (Eds): *Goodman and Gilman's The Pharmacological Basis of Therapeutics*, 7th Ed. New York, Macmillan, 1985, p. 266, with permission.)

373. Skeletal muscle

374. Lung and blood

375. Fat

Questions 376–378: Figure 9 shows distribution of thiopental in different body tissues and organs following its intravenous injection.

376. Skeletal muscle and skin

377. Adipose tissue

378. Brain, heart, liver, and kidneys

DIRECTIONS (Questions 379–383): The set of lettered headings below is followed by a list of numbered words and phrases. For each numbered word or phrase select

   A if the item is associated with **A** only
   B if the item is associated with **B** only
   C if the item is associated with both **A** and **B**
   D if the item is associated with neither **A** nor **B**

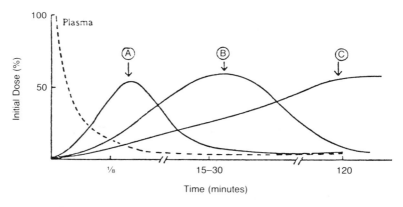

Figure 9 (Reproduced from Price HL, et al: The uptake of thiopental by body tissues and its relation to the duration of narcosis. *Clin Pharmacol Ther* 1960; 1:16–22, with permission.)

Questions 379–383:

    A. Nitrous oxide
    B. Enflurane

379. Produces some neuromuscular blockade during anesthesia

380. Produces a mild stimulation of salivary secretion

381. Sensitizes the myocardium to catecholamines

382. Lacks the potency when used alone for deep surgical anesthesia

383. Produces bradycardia especially during induction

DIRECTIONS (Questions 384–391): For each of the questions or incomplete statements below, **one** or **more** of the answers or completions given is correct. Select
    A if only 1, 2, and 3 are correct
    B if only 1 and 3 are correct
    C if only 2 and 4 are correct
    D if only 4 is correct
    E if all are correct

---

384. The principal factors that determine the acceptability of an agent for use as a general anesthetic are
    1. rapid and pleasant induction of, and recovery from, anesthesia
    2. a wide margin of safety
    3. adequate relaxation of skeletal muscles
    4. the absence of adverse effects in the amount used

		Directions Summarized		
A	**B**	**C**	**D**	**E**
1,2,3	1,3	2,4	4	All are
only	only	only	only	correct

385. The ease with which the most widely used inhalation anesthetics produce induction of anesthesia depends on
  1. the potency of the agent
  2. the vapor pressure at $20°C$
  3. the blood: gas partition coefficient
  4. the oil: gas partition coefficient

386. The anesthetic agent halothane
  1. reduces stroke volume of the heart and systemic blood pressure
  2. stimulates the sympathetic nervous system
  3. slows the heart rate during anesthesia
  4. has an irritant effect on the tracheobronchial tree

387. The intravenous anesthetic ketamine induces a state termed dissociative anesthesia which includes
  1. postanesthetic vivid dreams
  2. preanesthetic vivid dreams
  3. postanesthetic disorientation
  4. postanesthetic sensory illusions

388. The intravenous anesthetic thiopental
  1. is a potent depressant of respiration
  2. lowers the respiratory response to increased plasma carbon dioxide
  3. generally does not increase intracranial pressure
  4. reversibly increases hepatic blood flow

389. Proposed central nervous system (CNS) neurotransmitters include which of the following:
  1. acetylcholine
  2. dopamine
  3. norepinephrine
  4. endorphins

390. Pharmacokinetic properties of an inhaled anesthetic include which of the following:
   1. concentration of anesthetic inhaled
   2. solubility of anesthetic in the blood
   3. rate of pulmonary blood flow
   4. rate of anesthetic metabolism

391. Inhaled anesthetics have which of the following effects on the brain?
   1. Decreases the metabolic rate
   2. Increases the metabolic rate
   3. Increases the cerebral blood flow
   4. Decreases the cerebral blood flow

Local Anesthetics

DIRECTIONS (Questions 392–401): Each of the questions or incomplete statements below is followed by five suggested answers or completions. Select the **one** that is best in each case.

392. The speed of nerve blockade by local anesthetics depends on all of the following factors EXCEPT
   A. whether myelinated or nonmyelinated neurons
   B. whether small or large neurons
   C. whether B, C, or A fibers
   D. whether sensory or motor neurons
   E. whether for pain or tactile conduction

393. The central nervous system effects of intravenous local anesthetics are as follows EXCEPT
   A. light-headedness
   B. restlessness
   C. tremors
   D. nystagmus with high blood levels
   E. miosis

394. Each of the following statements is true for local anesthetics EXCEPT
   A. the ester type such as procaine and tetracaine are degraded principally by the liver
   B. the ester type are metabolized to *p*-aminobenzoic acid
   C. local anesthetics may cause asthmatic attacks in hypersensitive individuals
   D. allergic dermatitis has been reported
   E. allergic reactions are more likely to occur in the ester type than in the amide type

395. When given intravenously, local anesthetics, except cocaine, usually have all of the following effects EXCEPT
   A. reduced electrical excitability
   B. decreased conduction rate
   C. reduced cardiac contractile strength
   D. vasoconstriction
   E. vasodilation

396. All of the following statements concerning local anesthetics are true EXCEPT
   A. increasing the calcium concentration to an isolated nerve potentiates the blocking action
   B. blockade results from preventing the elevated increase in the permeability of the excited membrane to sodium
   C. diazepam is the preferred drug for treating the convulsion caused by local anesthetics
   D. the ester type are hydrolyzed in the blood at a rapid rate
   E. drowsiness is the most common symptom of a CNS effect

397. All of the following statements concerning local anesthetics are true EXCEPT
   A. generally available as the slightly acid hydrochloride
   B. greater stability as an acid salt rather than a free base
   C. a resting nerve is easier to block than one recently stimulated
   D. those with faster rates of degradation are safer
   E. when respiratory arrest occurs during spinal anesthesia, the most likely cause is ischemia of the medullary center

398. The major mechanism of action of local anesthetics involves

    A. an increase in the surface pressure of the lipid layer making up the nerve membrane, and thereby closing the pores through which ions move

    B. changes in permeability by increasing the degree of disorder of the membrane

    C. physical obstruction of the membrane sodium channel by combining with a specific receptor site in that channel

    D. alteration of the kinetics of opening of the sodium channel by calcium

    E. a reduction in permeability of resting nerve membrane to potassium and sodium ions

399. Which of the following statements is true of cocaine?

    A. Its local vasoconstrictor acts to limit its absorption, so that it can be applied to mucous membranes for surface anesthesia without fear of systemic toxicity

    B. Its central stimulating action is manifested first on the medullary respiratory center

    C. It blocks both the excitatory and inhibitory responses of sympathetically innervated organs to epinephrine, norepinephrine, and sympathetic nerve stimulation

    D. Its most important clinical action is its ability to block nerve conduction when applied topically; its most striking systemic effect is CNS stimulation

    E. It is not metabolized by the liver and depends on urinary excretion for its elimination from the body

400. Each of the following statements is true regarding the cardiovascular effects of local anesthetic agents EXCEPT
  A. high systemic concentrations block cardiac sodium channels and depress conduction excitability of the heart
  B. the effects on threshold and conduction time may depend on the presence of the cationic form in the extracellular medium
  C. a decrease in myocardial contractile strength and a reduction in blood pressure occur
  D. the primary action is on the myocardium
  E. inadvertently injected intravenously, it has produced ventricular fibrillation

401. Each of the following statements is true concerning spinal anesthesia with local anesthetics EXCEPT
  A. the drug concentration in the cerebral spinal fluid is lowered rapidly after its injection
  B. the somatic fibers for pain are anesthetized at a higher cephalic level than are the sympathetic fibers
  C. cerebrospinal fluid contains very little esterase and contributes little to degradation of the local anesthetic
  D. side effects are mainly those associated with sympathetic blockade
  E. the loss of tone in veins and venules are the most important change in the cardiovascular system

---

DIRECTIONS (Questions 402–404): The group of questions below consists of five lettered headings followed by a list of numbered phrases or statements. For each numbered phrase or statement, select the **one** lettered heading that is most closely associated with it. Each lettered heading may be selected once, more than once, or not at all.

Questions 402–404:

  A. Tetracaine
  B. Prilocaine
  C. Mepivacaine
  D. Bupivacaine
  E. Etidocaine

402. A local anesthetic of the amide type which may produce methemoglobinemia as a unique toxic after-effect

403. Long-acting derivative of lidocaine

404. A *p*-aminobenzoic acid ester producing a longer acting local anesthetic effect than that produced by procaine

Skeletal Muscle Relaxants and Neuromuscular-Blocking Drugs

DIRECTIONS (Questions 405–415): Each set of lettered headings below is followed by a list of numbered words and phrases. For each numbered word or phrase select

    A if the item is associated with **A** only
    B if the item is associated with **B** only
    C if the item is associated with both **A** and **B**
    D if the item is associated with neither **A** nor **B**

Questions 405–410:

    A. Tubocurarine chloride
    B. Succinylcholine chloride
    C. Both
    D. Neither

405. A single intravenous dose of 10 to 30 mg usually produces muscle paralysis of only 5 minute duration

406. Abnormal variant with low pseudocholinesterase activity which leads to prolonged duration of activity

407. Exerts its effects through an initial depolarization of the motor end-plate in skeletal muscle, which may be manifested as transient muscle fasciculation

408. Its neuromuscular blocking effects can be antagonized by an anticholinesterase drug such as neostigmine

409. A recent drug, atracurium (Tracrium), is a rapidly metabolized nondepolarizing drug similar in action to one of the above drugs

410. May increase both the intraocular and intragastric pressures

Questions 411–415:

    A. Dantrolene sodium
    B. Baclofen
    C. Both
    D. Neither

411. Used in the treatment of the rare malignant hyperthermia

412. One of the adverse effects of this drug is muscle weakness

413. Does not affect neuromuscular transmission nor does it change the electrical properties of skeletal muscle membranes

414. An active muscle relaxant that acts as a γ-aminobutyric acid agonist at the GABA-b receptors

415. A muscle relaxant with a mechanism of action directly on the skeletal muscle

Sedatives and Hypnotics

DIRECTIONS (Questions 416–418): Each of the questions or incomplete statements below is followed by five suggested answers or completions. Select the **one** that is best in each case.

416. This class of drugs, when used in high doses for long periods of time
   A. may be manifested as a generalized depressive at all effective dose levels
   B. may produce tolerance to the sedative-hypnotic effect
   C. does not lead to cross tolerance with the other sedatives
   D. may be life threatening even at small doses
   E. will irreversibly alter the endoplasmic reticular system of the cells

417. The sedative-hypnotic drug methaqualone, which has experienced widespread abuse in recent years, has each of the following properties EXCEPT
   A. its effects have been likened by users to those of heroin, producing a dissociative high and aphrodisiac activity
   B. it appears to lack significant analgesic activity, but enhances the effect of codeine
   C. it possesses anticonvulsant, anticholinergic, local anesthetic, antihistaminic, and antitussive activity
   D. it might be considered for clinical use in patients who have had unsatisfactory results with other hypnotics as it is devoid of ability to depress REM sleep
   E. continued ingestion in doses greater than therapeutic dose may lead to severe psychologic and physical dependence

418. Which one of the following drugs is not a benzodiazepine?
   A. Prazepam (Centrax)
   B. Triazolam (Halcion)
   C. Temazepam (Restoral)
   D. Gluethimide (Doriden)
   E. Alprazolam (Xanax)

DIRECTIONS (Questions 419–424): For each of the questions or incomplete statements below, **one** or **more** of the answers or completions given is correct. Select
   A if only 1, 2, and 3 are correct
   B if only 1 and 3 are correct
   C if only 2 and 4 are correct
   D if only 4 is correct
   E if all are correct

Directions Summarized				
A	**B**	**C**	**D**	**E**
1,2,3	1,3	2,4	4	All are
only	only	only	only	correct

419. Concerning tolerance and the sedative-hypnotic drugs, which of the following statements is (are) correct?
   1. Cross tolerance may lead to less effect by the other sedative-hypnotic drugs
   2. Abstinence convulsions may occur
   3. Addicts manifest a compulsion to take these drugs and to increase the dose
   4. Most of these drugs have a very long duration of action

420. Regarding sleep induced by oral administration of short-acting barbiturates such as secobarbital
   1. it appears to result from a selective action on the reticular-activating system
   2. the time spent in REM (paradoxical) sleep is reduced
   3. the hypnotic action usually requires 30 to 60 minutes for its onset
   4. sleep is usually maintained uninterrupted for 5 to 6 hours

421. In addition to an increased incidence of stillbirths and spontaneous abortions due to excessive drinking, in recent years a fetal alcohol syndrome has been described which consists of
   1. impairment of growth rate
   2. a characteristic cluster of facial abnormalities
   3. extensive impairment of the immune system
   4. fatty infiltration of the liver and other hepatic disorders

422. The benzodiazepine derivatives such as loraxepam and prazepam, among others, are generally classified as antianxiety drugs. However, they do
1. possess sedative properties but only weak hypnotic effects
2. lack the marked taming effect of the carbamates on spontaneously aggressive animals
3. display marked anticonvulsant activity and appear to restrict the spread of spontaneous generalized seizure activity as well as suppress drug-induced EEG epileptiform activity
4. have only a slight capacity for skeletal muscle relaxation, except indirectly as a result of their sedative action

423. Of the following group of benzodiazepine derivatives, those agents classified as hypnotic drugs rather than antianxiety agents are
1. halazepam (Paxipam)
2. alprazolam (Xanax)
3. clonazepam (Klonopin)
4. temazepam (Restoril)

424. The most frequent drug interaction involving the sedative-hypnotic is
1. blood loss due to interference with the anticoagulants
2. increased intraocular pressure when used with general anesthetics
3. blockade of the effect of the benzodiazepines
4. cross tolerance with other CNS-depressant drugs

Anticonvulsants

DIRECTIONS (Questions 425–428): Each of the questions or incomplete statements below is followed by five suggested answers or completions. Select the **one** that is best in each case.

425. Which of the following anticonvulsants is first used to treat partial seizures, often in generalized tonic-clonic seizures, and in some patients with trigeminal neuralgia?
  A. Carbamazepine
  B. Ethosuximide
  C. Valproic acid
  D. Diazepam
  E. Phenobarbital

426. Which of the following anticonvulsants is most often used to treat absence (petit mal) seizures?
  A. Ethosuximide
  B. Phenobarbital
  C. Carbamazepine
  D. Bromide
  E. Diazepam

427. Most antiepileptic drugs act by
  A. dilation of blood vessels only at site of seizure focus
  B. constriction of blood vessels in the brain
  C. prevention of excessive discharge from seizure focus
  D. prevention of activation of normal neurons at the seizure site
  E. increase in inhibitory impulses

428. Children who have experienced a convulsion associated with a febrile illness have an increased risk of becoming epileptic. If anticonvulsant therapy of the child is indicated, the drug of choice is
  A. phenobarbital
  B. diazepam
  C. secobarbital
  D. phenytoin
  E. clonazepam

DIRECTIONS (Questions 429–431): The group of questions below consists of five lettered headings followed by a list of numbered phrases or statements. For each numbered phrase or statement, select the **one** lettered heading that is most closely associated with it. Each lettered heading may be selected once, more than once, or not at all.

Questions 429–431:

    A. Valproic acid
    B. Primidone
    C. Phenytoin
    D. Clonazepam
    E. Carbamazepine

429. An iminostilbene derivative structurally related to the tricyclic antidepressants which is particularly effective in treatment of partial seizures with complex symptomatology

430. Useful in treatment of absence seizures but has its greatest usefulness as a sole agent given intravenously for status epilepticus

431. First drug discovered that does not cause sedation and yet is effective in controlling epileptic seizures

Analgesics and Antipyretics

DIRECTIONS (Questions 432–440): Each group of questions below consists of five lettered headings followed by a list of numbered words, phrases, or statements. For each numbered word, phrase, or statement, select the **one** lettered heading that is most closely associated with it. Each lettered heading may be selected once, more than once, or not at all.

Questions 432–436:

    A. Sodium salicylate
    B. Acetylcysteine
    C. Colchicine
    D. Acetaminophen
    E. Sulfinpyrazone

432. Effective in the treatment of gout by inhibition of the movement of leukocytes into the inflamed joint

433. Inhibits the synthesis of prostaglandins

434. A. Edward, a 51-year-old man weighing approximately 65
kg, after consuming several bottles of beer during the course
of an evening, drank the entire contents of two 8-ounce
bottles of **Brand Name** (adult liquid pain reliever), called
drug A, at about 10 PM. At breakfast time, around 8 AM the
following day, he experienced anorexia, nausea, vomiting,
and abdominal pain. At the insistence of his wife, he agreed
to see a physician. A serum assay revealed a plasma concentration of **drug A** greater than 70 μg/mL. A 5% solution
of **drug B** was given as a loading dose of 180 mL (140
mg/kg). The patient was then admitted to the hospital
where administration of **drug B** was continued in doses of
90 mL of the 5% solution at 4-hour intervals until assays
indicated that **drug A** concentration in plasma was below
hepatotoxic levels.

435. Drug A, the agent producing the toxic effects

436. Drug B, the agent used to antagonize the toxic effects of
drug A

Questions 437–440:

    A. Mefenamic acid (Ponstel)
    B. Diflunisal (Dolobid)
    C. Meclofenamate sodium (Meclomen)
    D. Ibuprofen (Motrin, Rufen)
    E. Tolmetin sodium (Tolectin)

437. Used clinically for the relief of mild to moderate pain when
therapy will not exceed 1 week

438. An acetic acid derivative with analgesic, antipyretic, and
anti-inflammatory properties, which is indicated for relief
of signs and symptoms of rheumatoid arthritis and osteoarthritis and is recommended for treatment of juvenile
rheumatoid arthritis

439. A recently available nonsteroidal anti-inflammatory drug
indicated for relief of signs and symptoms of acute and
chronic rheumatoid arthritis and osteoarthritis

440. A salicylic acid derivative three to four times more potent than aspirin as an analgesic in treatment of osteoarthritis and musculoskeletal strains or pains

---

DIRECTIONS (Questions 441–445): The set of lettered headings below is followed by a list of numbered words or phrases. For each numbered word or phrase select

    A if the item is associated with **A** only
    B if the item is associated with **B** only
    C if the item is associated with both **A** and **B**
    D if the item is associated with neither **A** nor **B**

Questions 441–445:

    A. Acetylsalicylic acid
    B. Probenecid
    C. Both
    D. Neither

441. Has both an analgesic effect and a uricosuric effect when given in doses of 1 g/day or less

442. Has been used in the treatment of gout

443. Should not be given to children and teenagers during or while recovering from chickenpox or influenza

444. Oral doses may cause gastric irritation and may even cause gastrointestinal bleeding

445. May interfere with the excretion of weak acids such as benzoic acid

DIRECTIONS (Questions 446–448): For each of the questions or incomplete statements below, **one** or **more** of the answers or completions given is correct. Select

A   if only 1, 2, and 3 are correct
B   if only 1 and 3 are correct
C   if only 2 and 4 are correct
D   if only 4 is correct
E   if all are correct

446. The analgesic action of salicylates is the result of
 1. their peripheral effect
 2. their cortical effect
 3. their hypothalamic effect
 4. lowering of the irritability of the reticular pathways

447. During mild chronic salicylate toxicity the patient can be expected to experience
 1. nausea and possibly vomiting
 2. vertigo
 3. tinnitus
 4. reduced auditory acuity

448. In severe aspirin toxicity in children, subsequent to stage of compensated respiratory alkalosis, there develops
 1. respiratory acidosis
 2. compensated acidosis
 3. metabolic acidosis
 4. uncompensated alkalosis

Narcotics

DIRECTIONS (Questions 449–466): Each of the questions or incomplete statements below is followed by five suggested answers or completions. Select the **one** that is best in each case.

449. All of the following are narcotics EXCEPT
   A. morphine
   B. codeine
   C. fentanyl
   D. meperidine
   E. all of the above

450. Each of the following is an action shared by all of the opioid analgesics EXCEPT
   A. depression of the respiratory center
   B. adequate absorption when given orally
   C. release of histamine
   D. depression of the cough reflex
   E. tendency to dry secretions

451. Opioid analgesics include all of the following EXCEPT
   A. opiates derived from opium
   B. opiopeptides such as enkephalins
   C. synthetic compounds related to the opium alkaloids
   D. morphine
   E. doxepin

452. Each of the following statements is true concerning the nausea resulting from morphine administration EXCEPT
   A. it results from stimulation of the chemoreceptor trigger zone for emesis
   B. it occurs in approximately 40% of the ambulatory patients
   C. it is counteracted by morphine antagonists
   D. it is unique in that codeine in equianalgesic doses does not cause nausea
   E. it is partly due, in ambulatory patients, to an increase in vestibular sensitivity

453. All of the following substances are present in opium EXCEPT
   A. codeine
   B. thebaine
   C. morphine
   D. cycazocine
   E. papaverine

454. All of the following are organ system effects of the narcotic analgesics EXCEPT
    A. euphoria
    B. respiratory depression
    C. emesis
    D. constipation
    E. myopia

455. Each of the following statements is true in relation to high biliary pressure caused in some patients by morphine EXCEPT
    A. results from spasm of the biliary tract
    B. results from increased tone of the sphincter of Oddi is prevented by morphine antagonists
    C. is frequently accompanied by elevated serum lipase and serum amylase
    D. is completely relieved by atropine
    E. is relieved by opioid antagonists

456. Each of the findings listed is characteristic of opioid poisoning EXCEPT
    A. coma
    B. pinpoint pupils
    C. depressed respiration
    D. flaccidity of skeletal muscles
    E. elevated body temperature

457. Morphine has all of the effects listed EXCEPT
    A. produces hyperglycemia
    B. decreases the release of thyroid stimulating hormone (TSH)
    C. decreases the release of thyroid hormone
    D. increases glucagon release by its action on the pancreas
    E. stimulates release of catecholamines from the adrenal medulla

458. In equianalgesic doses, methadone and morphine are equal in each of the following effects EXCEPT
   A. analgesic potency
   B. antitussive action
   C. duration of analgesic action
   D. degree of respiratory depression
   E. miosis

459. Each of the following is an acceptable and satisfactory method for overcoming addiction to opioids EXCEPT
   A. administration of clonidine and methadone
   B. acute withdrawal
   C. a gradual daily reduction of the dose until no drug is being given
   D. substituting methadone for morphine or heroin and then reducing the dose of methadone by 50% every other day
   E. shifting the addict onto a methadone maintenance program

460. From 1 to 7 days after withdrawal of short-acting barbiturates, dependent individuals may manifest convulsions, hallucinations, and each of the following effects EXCEPT
   A. vomiting
   B. hypotension and tachycardia
   C. fever
   D. coarse tremors
   E. sedation and sleepiness

461. Each of the following statements concerning the endogenous brain peptides with opiatelike activity is true EXCEPT

A. there is evidence for at least four types of receptors for these peptides and opioid drugs in the brain and other organs, designated mu, kappa, delta, and sigma

B. many synthetic congeners with preferential affinities for certain drug types of receptors have been prepared; these have been proved to be relatively selective agonists

C. three distinct families of these peptides, the enkephalins, the endorphins, and the dynorphins, are presently known to exist

D. each opioid family is derived from a genetically distinct precursor polypeptide, which also contains a number of biologically inactive peptides present exclusively in brain tissue

E. they appear to function as neurotransmitters, modulators of neurotransmission, or as neurohormones

462. The analgesic effect of morphine and other opioids may be enhanced and the sedative effect simultaneously diminished by combining with the narcotic drug a small dose of

A. levallorphan

B. amphetamine

C. dextromethorphan

D. naltrexone

E. noscapine

463. Each of the following statements is true of meperidine, the prototype of the phenylpiperidine opioid analgesics, EXCEPT

A. it was introduced into therapy as an antispasmodic of the atropine type

B. heart rate is not significantly affected by intramuscular administration, but intravenous doses often result in tachycardia

C. it differs from morphine in that toxic doses sometimes cause overt manifestations of CNS excitation

D. it has respiratory depressant actions that are not antagonized by naloxone

E. its adverse effects are similar to those occurring with equianalgesic doses of morphine except for less frequent constipation and urinary retention

464. Morphine can be used in all of the following conditions EXCEPT

A. persistent cough

B. acute pulmonary edema

C. anesthetic premedication where adverse postoperative effects are undesirable

D. diarrhea

E. for pain in patients with terminal cancer

465. Which of the following drugs may be used as a narcotic antagonist?

A. Proproxyphene

B. Fentanyl

C. Naloxone

D. Meperidine

E. Naltrexone

466. The use of narcotic analgesics may result in all of the following effects EXCEPT

A. decrease in urine output

B. tolerance

C. stimulate the release of prolactin

D. stimulate the release of antidiuretic hormone

E. mydriasis and myopia

DIRECTIONS (Questions 467–469 (Figure 10)): Select the correct formula for each of the following drugs:

467. Morphine

468. Codeine

469. Naloxone (narcotic antagonist)

Central Nervous System Stimulants

DIRECTIONS (Questions 470–477): Each set of lettered headings below is followed by a list of numbered words or phrases. For each numbered word or phrase select

    A if the item is associated with **A** only
    B if the item is associated with **B** only
    C if the item is associated with both **A** and **B**
    D if the item is associated with neither **A** nor **B**

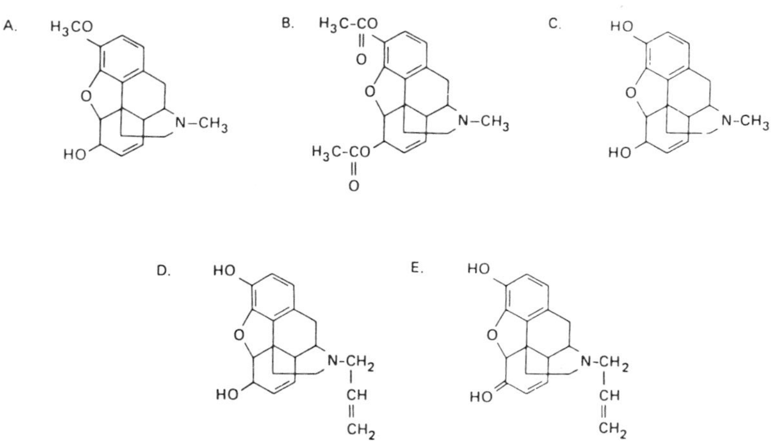

Figure 10

Questions 470-473:

    A. Pentylenetetrazol
    B. Methylphenidate
    C. Both
    D. Neither

470. Has mild CNS stimulant effects which are more pronounced on mental than on motor activities

471. Useful in emergency treatment of individuals who are severely intoxicated by general CNS depressants

472. Used to treat children with hyperkinetic syndrome

473. Similar action as amphetamine with the same abuse potential

Questions 474-477:

    A. Theophylline
    B. Caffeine
    C. Both
    D. Neither

474. Present in coffee at about 100 mg/cup

475. Side effects in treatment of asthma are nervousness and tremors

476. Most effective bronchodilator of the methylxanthines

477. Focal and generalized convulsions have occurred in patients when the blood concentration was only about 50% above the upper limit of the accepted therapeutic range

Drugs Affecting Behavior

DIRECTIONS (Questions 478–487): Each of the questions or incomplete statements below is followed by five suggested answers or completions. Select the **one** that is best in each case.

478. The earliest and longest lasting effect of lysergic acid diethyl-amide (LSD) is
    A. insomnia
    B. pupillary dilation
    C. hyperreflexia of the masseter muscles
    D. elevation of body temperature
    E. tachycardia with accompanying increase in blood pressure

479. The development of the current antipsychotic drugs is an outgrowth of research on
    A. atropine substitutes
    B. antianxiety drugs
    C. antihistamines
    D. sedative-hypnotic drugs
    E. antiemetics

480. Among the data supporting a role of dopamine antagonism in the therapeutic action of antipsychotic drugs are all of the following findings EXCEPT
    A. they increase the rate of production of dopamine metabolism in the midbrain
    B. small doses block behavioral and neuroendocrine effects of dopamine agonists
    C. they inhibit a dopamine-sensitive adenylate cyclase system in homogenates of caudate or limbic tissue
    D. inhibition of tyrosine hydroxylase, the rate-limiting enzyme in catecholamine biosynthesis, in schizophrenic patients allows marked reduction of dose of these drugs
    E. drugs such as amphetamines, which block dopamine uptake at brain receptor sites, reduce symptoms of schizophrenia

481. Adverse effects of antipsychotic drugs include all of the following EXCEPT
  A. dry mouth
  B. Parkinson's syndrome
  C. infertility
  D. sinus arrhythmias
  E. drowsiness

482. The antipsychotic drugs are divided into the following chemical or drug classes EXCEPT
  A. heterocyclic compounds
  B. phenothiazine
  C. amphetamine
  D. thioxanthene
  E. butyrophenone

483. The antipsychotic agents may produce adverse effects, which include all of those listed below EXCEPT
  A. psychoses in nonpsychotic subjects
  B. tardive dyskinesia
  C. impotence
  D. akathisia
  E. none of the above

484. The endocrine system is affected by the antipsychotic drugs leading to all of the following adverse effects EXCEPT
  A. gynecomastia in men
  B. amenorrhea
  C. dystonia
  D. galactorrhea
  E. false-positive pregnancy test

485. The "second-generation antidepressants" include all of the following EXCEPT
  A. amoxapine (Asendin)
  B. trazodone (Desyrel)
  C. maprotiline (Ludiomil)
  D. amintripyline (Elavil)
  E. fluoxetine (Prozac)

486. Categories of antidepressant drugs are as follows EXCEPT
  A. tricyclic tertiary amines
  B. second-generation
  C. dopaminergic inhibitor
  D. monoamine inhibitor
  E. tricyclic secondary amines

487. The development of the current antipsychotic drugs is an outgrowth of research on
  A. atropine substitutes
  B. antianxiety drugs
  C. antihistamines
  D. sedative-hypnotic drugs
  E. antiemetics

DIRECTIONS (Questions 488–504): Each group of questions below consists of five lettered headings followed by a list of numbered words, phrases, or statements. For each numbered word, phrase, or statement, select the **one** lettered heading that is most closely associated with it. Each lettered heading may be selected once, more than once, or not at all.

Questions 488–493:

  A. Loxapine (Loxitane)
  B. Amoxapine (Asendin)
  C. Trazodone (Desyrel)
  D. Molindone (Moban)
  E. Haloperidol (Haldol)

488. An antidepressant agent chemically unrelated to tricyclic, tetracyclic, or other known antidepressant drugs

489. Representative of a new class of tricyclic antipsychotic agents chemically distinct from the thioxanthenes, butyrophenones, and phenothiazines

490. A dihydroindolone classified as an antipsychotic drug with a primary indication for treating schizophrenics

491. An antipsychotic drug which is very useful in situations where sedation and hypotension is undesirable

492. A second-generation antidepressant drug with a mild sedation component to its action

493. A butyrophenone antipsychotic drug with severe extrapyramidal adverse effect

Questions 494–497:

    A. Tranylcypromine (Parnate)
    B. Amitriptyline (Elavil)
    C. Thioridazine (Mellaril)
    D. Clozapine (Clozanil)
    E. Haloperidol (Haldol)

494. Low incidence of extrapyramidal syndrome

495. May cause a small incidence of serious agranulocytosis

496. A tricyclic antidepressant drug

497. A monoamine oxidase (MAO) inhibitor used as an antidepressant drug

Questions 498–500:

    A. Clomiprimine (Anafranil)
    B. Isocarboxazid (Marplan)
    C. Imipramine (Tofranil)
    D. Methylphenidate (Ritalin)
    E. Lithium carbonate

498. Useful in treatment of retarded, endogenous, or possible psychotic depressions

499. Concomitant administration with a tricyclic antidepressant may result in increased plasma levels of the tricyclic

500. Tricyclic first-generation antidepressant drug

Questions 501–504:

    A. Tranylcypromine (Parnate)
    B. Meprobamate (Miltown)
    C. Chlordiazepoxide (Librium)
    D. Chlorpromazine (Thorazine)
    E. Mescaline

501. Widely used benzodiazepine antianxiety drug having central skeletal muscle-relaxing properties

502. Possesses two modes of action: potent inhibition of monoamine oxidase and an amphetaminelike action

503. May produce postural hypotension, which has generally been attributed to an α-adrenergic blocking action

504. The occurrence of acute hypertensive crisis with fatal subarachnoid hemorrhage after ingestion of certain foods led to a sharp curtailment of its use

---

DIRECTIONS (Questions 505–517): For each of the questions or incomplete statements below, **one** or **more** of the answers or completions given is correct. Select

    A if only 1, 2, and 3 are correct
    B if only 1 and 3 are correct
    C if only 2 and 4 are correct
    D if only 4 is correct
    E if all are correct

---

505. Among the autonomic nervous system effects of the phenothiazines is their ability to
    1. produce α-adrenoceptor blockade when given as a single small dose
    2. inhibit the uptake mechanism for catecholamines in adrenergic neuronal terminals in the central nervous system
    3. potentiate blood sugar responses to norepinephrine with chronic administration
    4. stimulate cholinergic muscarinic receptors at peripheral effector sites

506. Chlorpromazine related phenothiazine derivatives are useful therapeutic agents in the treatment of
1. psychoses
2. nausea and vomiting
3. intractable hiccup
4. motion sickness

507. The general characteristics of phenothiazines are that
1. they seem to act by depressing the vomiting center rather than the trigger zone
2. they possess α-adrenergic potentiating effects when given as a single dose
3. they enhance the nicotinic and muscarinic actions of acetylcholine
4. most of them possess significant antiemetic activity, making a wide choice of agents for this purpose possible

508. The influence of phenothiazines on neuroendocrine activity
1. is to inhibit release of growth hormone, perhaps by an action on the hypothalamus
2. can be manifested as a delay in ovulation during chlorpromazine therapy, apparently as a result of the hypothalamus interfering with pituitary gonadotropin output
3. may be manifested as amenorrhea, sometimes seen during therapy with large doses
4. is to depress the hypothalamus, thereby interfering with milk formation in lactating patients by inhibiting release of lactogenic hormone

509. Facts related to the toxicity of the phenothiazines are
1. approximately 40% of patients taking substituted phenothiazines show extrapyramidal symptoms
2. extrapyramidal symptoms with substituted phenothiazines include akathisia (motor restlessness), parkinsonism, and dyskinesia (dystonic reactions)
3. the extrapyramidal symptoms associated with phenothiazine therapy are not always reversible, even when treated with antiparkinsonism medication
4. with the phenothiazines, agranulocytosis is a frequently occurring irreversible complication

	Directions Summarized			
A	**B**	**C**	**D**	**E**
1,2,3	1,3	2,4	4	All are
only	only	only	only	correct

510. The phenothiazine derivative, thiethylperazine (Torecan)
    1. is currently marketed only as an antiemetic
    2. is a potent dopaminergic antagonist
    3. has many neurolepticlike properties
    4. in high doses is an effective antipsychotic drug

511. Among the findings concerning the effects of tricyclic antidepressants, based on their action on brain amines
    1. inhibition of neuronal uptake of dopamine seems to be associated with stimulant rather than antidepressant activity
    2. block of serotonin transport may result in both sedative and antidepressant effects
    3. blockade of norepinephrine uptake seems to correlate with antidepressant activity
    4. interference with transport of serotonin and norepinephrine into certain brain neurons seems to be the mechanism of action of these drugs

512. The use of lithium carbonate in the treatment of bipolar affective disorder may lead to which of the following adverse effects?
    1. Tremor and other neurologic effects
    2. Mental confusion and other psychiatric disturbances
    3. polydipsia and polyuria
    4. altered T wave leading to myocardial failure

513. Antipsychotic drugs alter the electroencephalographic frequencies pattern plus which other changes?
    1. May produce seizures in patients without a history of epilepsy
    2. The hypersynchrony (slowing) of the EEG may lead to a wrong diagnosis
    3. The EEG changes appear to start in the subcortical region of the brain
    4. The hypersynchrony starts in the hypothalamus region

514. Antipsychotic drugs may be used in a variety of conditions as listed below EXCEPT
1. opioid withdrawal syndrome
2. control of agitated state in senile dementia
3. control of psychosis or agitation in psychotic patients
4. relief of anxiety in normal subjects

515. Behavioral changes in patients using antipsychotic agents include
1. akinesia with mental depression
2. mental depression from overdoses
3. mental confusion from toxic overdoses
4. supersensitivity to drugs such as amphetamine

516. Nonpsychiatric uses of antipsychotic drugs include
1. mild sedation in normal subjects
2. antiemetic action in cancer therapy
3. hypnosis in normal subjects
4. antiemetic action after anesthesia

517. Lithium blood levels are monitored to
1. establish a maintenance dose
2. avoid toxic levels after delivery
3. detect lithium renal clearance increases during pregnancy
4. avoid skin rashes

Explanatory Answers

364. A. In contrast to anesthetic agents with high partition coefficients, anesthetic agents with low partition coefficients are relatively insoluble gases that readily leave the blood and enter the brain, leading to a rapid induction of surgical anesthesia. (**Ref.** 1, pp. 306–307; **Ref.** 2, pp. 452–543; **Ref.** 6, pp. 264, 277; **Ref.** 8, p. 482; **Ref.** 9, pp. 405–406)

365. C. The most frequent change in cardiac rhythm during methoxyflurane anesthesia is sinus bradycardia, which responds well to belladonna alkaloids. (**Ref.** 1, pp. 309–310; **Ref.** 2, pp. 463–465; **Ref.** 6, pp. 412, 506; **Ref.** 8, p. 297; **Ref.** 9, p. 416)

366. E. Diazepam is used to achieve anesthesia. Although the final depth of anesthesia is light, the recovery is slow and the patient will have a period of amnesia. (**Ref.** 1, pp. 305–306; **Ref.** 2, pp. 474–475; **Ref.** 8, pp. 303–305; **Ref.** 9, pp. 424–425)

367. E. Increased salivary secretion is seldom a problem during intravenous barbiturate anesthesia and constitutes an advantage of these agents. (**Ref.** 1, p. 322; **Ref.** 2, pp. 445, 473; **Ref.** 6, pp. 292–294; **Ref.** 8, pp. 301–303; **Ref.** 9, pp. 424–425)

368. C. Since the maximum allowable concentration (MAC) of methoxyflurane is only 0.16%, induction anesthesia can be achieved with inhaled concentrations of 2% to 3%; induction requires 20 to 30 minutes, however. (**Ref.** 1, p. 309; **Ref.** 2, pp. 463–467; **Ref.** 6, p. 288; **Ref.** 8, p. 286; **Ref.** 9, p. 419)

369. B. This excitatory action of enflurane is not thought to be of special concern, but the drug should be avoided in patients with seizure foci. (**Ref.** 1, p. 309; **Ref.** 2, p. 284; **Ref.** 6, p. 285; **Ref.** 8, p. 292; **Ref.** 9, p. 416)

370. D. Although blood pressure decreases with dose, cardiac output may increase markedly in response to hypercapnia with isoflurane anesthesia. (**Ref.** 1, pp. 309–310; **Ref.** 2, pp. 463–467; **Ref.** 6, p. 286; **Ref.** 8, p. 295; **Ref.** 9, p. 416)

371. E. Nitrous oxide is the one inhalation anesthetic that does not alter the heart or respiration when used with 15% to 20% oxygen. (**Ref.** 1, p. 309; **Ref.** 2, p. 284; **Ref.** 8, p. 299; **Ref.** 9, p. 417)

372. B. The brain, heart, and kidney are high blood-flow viscera to which significant amounts of anesthetic agents are delivered during its administration, resulting in gas tension increases and decreases in these tissues paralleling those in blood. (**Ref.** 1, pp. 311–312; **Ref.** 2, pp. 471–472; **Ref.** 6, pp. 265–266; **Ref.** 8, p. 274)

373. C. Although the tissue : blood partition coefficient of most anesthetic agents is near unity for many lean body tissues, the blood flow to muscle is relatively low so that equilibration of blood and tissue tensions is reached rather slowly. (**Ref.** 1, p. 311; **Ref.** 2, p. 471; **Ref.** 6, pp. 264–266; **Ref.** 8, p. 275)

374. A. With the first breath of anesthetic gas, the alveolar tension of nitrous oxide begins to increase and continues rapidly through the early uptake phase; the arterial tension of this gas reaches 90% of the inspired tension in about 20 minutes. (**Ref.** 1, p. 311; **Ref.** 2, p. 471; **Ref.** 6, pp. 262–266; **Ref.** 8, p. 298; **Ref.** 9, p. 407)

375. D. The relatively poor blood flow to adipose tissue results in a slow increase in nitrous oxide gas tension in fat, but because of the high tissue : blood coefficient for these tissues, its concentration in fatty tissue is much greater than that in blood at the time of equilibrium. (**Ref.** 1, p. 311; **Ref.** 2, p. 471; **Ref.** 6, pp. 265–266; **Ref.** 9, pp. 407–408)

376. B. Following initial distribution of thiopental to brain and other tissues with high blood flow, a relatively rapid redistribution of the drug occurs, principally to "indifferent" tissues with a large mass, such as muscle. (**Ref.** 1, p. 311; **Ref.** 2, p. 444; **Ref.** 6, p. 292; **Ref.** 9, p. 204)

377. C. Although thiopental penetrates all cells readily, it has an especially high affinity for fat. The delay in the peak concentration is due to the relatively poor blood supply to this tissue. (**Ref.** 1, p. 311; **Ref.** 2, p. 444; **Ref.** 9, p. 422)

378. A. The rapid entry of thiopental into the brain, liver, and kidneys is related to its high lipid solubility, and the short duration of the resulting anesthesia to its redistribution from the brain, which it enters rapidly. (**Ref.** 1, p. 311; **Ref.** 2, p. 444; **Ref.** 6, p. 292; **Ref.** 9, pp. 421–423)

379. B. The muscle relaxant activity of enflurane is caused by actions in both central nervous system and the skeletal neuromuscular junction. (**Ref.** 1, p. 311; **Ref.** 2, p. 436; **Ref.** 8, p. 293; **Ref.** 9, p. 416)

380. B. Although mild stimulation of salivation and respiratory secretions are caused by enflurane, these are not serious, and the use of muscarinic blocking agents is not usually necessary. (**Ref.** 1, pp. 311–312; **Ref.** 2, p. 437; **Ref.** 6, p. 283; **Ref.** 8, p. 292; **Ref.** 9, p. 416)

381. B. Nitrous oxide is devoid of sensitizing effect on the heart and enflurane's myocardial sensitizing effect is less than that of its chemical relative, halothane. (**Ref.** 1, p. 311; **Ref.** 2, p. 437; **Ref.** 6, p. 285; **Ref.** 8, p. 299; **Ref.** 9, p. 414)

382. A. Nitrous oxide, when used with 20% oxygen, lacks the potency to induce deep surgical anesthesia. It is combined with other anesthetic agents for this purpose. (**Ref.** 1, p. 309; **Ref.** 2, pp. 465–467; **Ref.** 8, p. 298; **Ref.** 9, p. 417)

383. D. Enflurane reduces the arterial blood pressure. While halothane induces bradycardia, enflurane will increase the heart rate. These cardiovascular effects are ameliorated by the use of preanesthetic medication, including atropine. (**Ref.** 1, p. 309; **Ref.** 2, p. 462; **Ref.** 8, pp. 287, 292; **Ref.** 9, p. 414)

384. C. Although all of these are characteristics of an ideal anesthetic agent, rapid induction may be achieved by use of ultrashort-acting barbiturates, and specific muscle relaxants may be used to relax skeletal muscle. (**Ref.** 1, p. 304; **Ref.** 2, p. 458; **Ref.** 6, p. 276; **Ref.** 9, pp. 420–421)

385. B. Potency expresses the tension, or partial pressure, required in the brain for anesthesia to occur. The blood:gas partition coefficient to the blood from the alveolar of vapor refers to that which must be transferred to the blood from the alveolar gas in order to achieve a given tension. (**Ref.** 1, p. 305; **Ref.** 2, pp. 460–462; **Ref.** 6, p. 277; **Ref.** 8, p. 285; **Ref.** 9, p. 402)

386. B. Halothane depresses the heart and circulation, but does not evoke a compensatory increase in sympathetic nervous system activity. (**Ref.** 1, p. 309; **Ref.** 2, p. 434; **Ref.** 8, p. 287; **Ref.** 9, p. 414)

387. A. Recovery from ketamine anesthesia can result in the "dissociative" state and this has limited the use of this drug. However, the amnesia has some advantages. Ketamine is used for short anesthesia. (**Ref.** 1, p. 312; **Ref.** 2, p. 476; **Ref.** 8, p. 306; **Ref.** 9, p. 425)

388. A. Thiopental is commonly used for short surgical procedures. It is also used to induce anesthesia. Due to respiratory and cardiovascular depression, this agent is not often used as the sole anesthetic for general anesthesia. (**Ref.** 1, p. 311; **Ref.** 2, pp. 473–474; **Ref.** 8, p. 303; **Ref.** 9, p. 423)

389. E. All of these chemicals plus a few others are considered CNS neurotransmitters. The CNS is so interconnected that it is difficult to establish directly any neurotransmitter. This leaves a lot of room to add new transmitters and to discard previously proposed transmitters. (**Ref.** 1, pp. 260–263; **Ref.** 2, pp. 438–440)

390. A. The inhaled anesthetics are metabolized to such a minor extent that this factor is not used in establishing the pharmacokinetic properties of these agents. (**Ref.** 1, pp. 306–308; **Ref.** 2, pp. 460–461; **Ref.** 8, p. 286)

391. B. While the metabolic rate of the brain slows during surgical anesthesia with the inhaled anesthetics, the cerebral blood flow increases. The latter may not be desirable where the patient has an elevated intracranial pressure since the pressure may increase further during inhalation anesthesia. (**Ref.** 1, p. 310; **Ref.** 2, pp. 462–463; **Ref.** 8, p. 288)

392. D. The smaller B and C fibers are blocked first followed by the A delta fibers. A number of surgical procedures are carried out under various local anesthesias such as spinal or epidural anesthesia, nerve block, and surface anesthesia. For the latter, tetracaine or lidocaine are preferred except for the nasopharynx, nose, and ear, where cocaine is preferred. (**Ref.** 1, pp. 318–319; **Ref.** 8, pp. 313, 322–325)

393. E. Local anesthetics are administered in such a way as to avoid tonic–clonic convulsions which result from high blood levels. The early signs of toxicity include light-headedness, restlessness, shivers, and rapid eye movements. With infiltration anesthesia, epinephrine may be added to reduce absorption of the local anesthetic; however, it should not be added where there are end arteries such as in fingers, toes, ears, nose, and penis. (**Ref.** 1, pp. 316–320; **Ref.** 6, p. 311; **Ref.** 8, pp. 317, 323)

394. A. The plasma pseudocholinesterase is mostly responsible for degrading the ester type of local anesthetics, though the liver contributes. The liberated products, especially PABA, have been implicated in the occasional allergic reactions. (**Ref.** 1, pp. 317, 321; **Ref.** 6, pp. 310–312; **Ref.** 8, pp. 318, 325; **Ref.** 9, pp. 430, 436)

395. D. The local anesthetics produce cardiovascular effects by their direct action on the heart and blood vessels and indirectly by acting on the autonomic nerves. Cocaine is the only one that causes vasoconstriction. (**Ref.** 1, p. 321; **Ref.** 6, p. 311; **Ref.** 8, p. 318; **Ref.** 9, p. 436)

396. A. The degree of blockade is reduced, not increased, as calcium levels are increased. Local anesthetics act by their direct interaction with voltage-sensitive Na^+ channels. (**Ref.** 8, p. 310)

397. C. A nerve recently stimulated is more easily blocked than a resting nerve. (**Ref.** 8, p. 316)

398. C. The proteins making up the mammalian sodium channel, apparently consisting of three dissimilar subunits of glycosylated proteins, have recently been purified on a large scale and constituted functionally. (**Ref.** 1, pp. 318–319; **Ref.** 6, pp. 303–304; **Ref.** 8, p. 312)

399. D. The marked stimulation, particularly of the cerebral cortex by cocaine, has helped to limit its uses to topical anesthesia for which other effective and less toxic drugs are now available. (**Ref.** 6, p. 309; **Ref.** 8, p. 319; **Ref.** 9, pp. 436–437)

400. A. Although the cardiovascular effects are usually seen only in the presence of high systemic concentrations of the drug, on rare occasions small (therapeutic) amounts will cause cardiovascular collapse and death. (**Ref.** 1, pp. 317–319; **Ref.** 6, p. 307; **Ref.** 8, p. 318; **Ref.** 9, p. 436)

401. B. Preganglionic sympathetic fibers are more sensitive to local anesthetic action than are the somatic sensory or motor fibers, thus the level of sympathetic denervation during hyperbaric spinal anesthesia extends an average of two spinal segments cephalad to the level of sensory anesthesia. (**Ref.** 6, p. 315; **Ref.** 8, pp. 322–324)

402. B. Prilocaine has pharmacologic properties similar to those of lidocaine but has a longer onset and duration of action. (**Ref.** 1, p. 316; **Ref.** 6, p. 311; **Ref.** 9, pp. 438–439)

403. E. The time required for production of anesthesia with etidocaine is about the same as for lidocaine but its anesthetic action lasts two to three times longer. (**Ref.** 1, p. 316; **Ref.** 6, p. 311; **Ref.** 9, p. 438)

404. A. Tetracaine is about 10 times more toxic and more active than procaine after intravenous injection. (**Ref.** 1, p. 316; **Ref.** 9, p. 437)

405. B. The extremely brief duration of action of succinylcholine is due principally to its inactivation by butyrylcholinesterase, the pseudocholinesterase of liver and plasma. (**Ref.** 6, pp. 229, 232; **Ref.** 9, pp. 213–214)

406. B. The duration of action of succinylcholine may be extended from minutes to hours in patients with low pseudocholinesterase activity. (**Ref.** 1, p. 326; **Ref.** 9, pp. 213–214)

407. B. Succinylcholine interacts with the cholinergic receptor at the end-plate to first stimulate, then produce, a two-phase block, resulting in flaccid paralysis. (**Ref.** 2, pp. 237–239; **Ref.** 4, p. 238; **Ref.** 6, pp. 226–228; **Ref.** 8, p. 171; **Ref.** 9, p. 213)

408. A. Drugs such as neostigmine and edrophonium, by virtue of their ability to both preserve acetylcholine and directly stimulate the neuromuscular junction, can overcome competitive blockade of acetylcholine receptors. The action of succinylcholine, particularly in its initial phase of action, would be accentuated by these drugs. (**Ref.** 6, p. 230)

409. A. This recent nondepolarizing drug, atracurium is of short duration due to rapid metabolism. The mechanism of action is like that of tubocurarine. (**Ref.** 1, p. 236; **Ref.** 9, p. 217)

410. B. Succinylcholine may increase both the intraocular and intragastric pressures. During ocular surgery the intraocular pressure change is of concern. The increased intragastric pressure could lead to expulsion of stomach contents during surgery. (**Ref.** 1, p. 329; **Ref.** 9, p. 214)

411. A. Malignant hyperthermia is triggered by a variety of stimuli including anesthesia. (**Ref.** 1, p. 333; **Ref.** 8, p. 176)

412. C. Both agents have the capacity to cause muscle weakness and this represents the most common major side effect of dantrolene. (**Ref.** 1, p. 333; **Ref.** 6, pp. 486–488; **Ref.** 8, pp. 479–481; **Ref.** 9, p. 218)

413. A. Dantrolene reduces contractions of skeletal muscle by a direct action on excitation–contraction coupling, perhaps by increasing the amount a calcium released from the sarcoplasmic reticulum. (**Ref.** 1, p. 332; **Ref.** 6, p. 488; **Ref.** 8, pp. 480–481; **Ref.** 9, p. 218)

414. B. Baclofen is *p*-chlorophenylGABA and it retains the actions of GABA at the GABA-b receptors. (**Ref.** 8, pp. 479–480; **Ref.** 9, p. 217)

415. A. Dantrolene appears to have a direct action on excitation–contraction coupling of skeletal muscle. (**Ref.** 1, p. 332; **Ref.** 6, p. 488; **Ref.** 8, pp. 480–481; **Ref.** 9, p. 218)

416. D. Although barbiturates do depress all brain cells, the action on ascending conduction in the reticular activating system appears to be selective and thus accounts for the major therapeutic usefulness of these compounds to produce sleep without causing significant depression of other functions. (**Ref.** 2, p. 505; **Ref.** 3, p. 289; **Ref.** 8, p. 359; **Ref.** 9, p. 449)

417. D. Even with its high abuse potential, methaqualone remains among the acceptable sedative-hypnotic drugs and may be used as such although there seems to be no basis for expecting results different from those produced by more well-established drugs. (**Ref.** 2, p. 511)

418. D. The benzodiazepines have names ending in pam or lam except chlordiazepoxide. Gluethimide is a sedative-hypnotic but not a benzodiazepine. (**Ref.** 1, pp. 365–366; **Ref.** 8, p. 347; **Ref.** 9, p. 446)

419. A. As the dose of a barbiturate is increased, habituation changes into addiction, in which the drug becomes a major part of the individual's life. Neither chlorpromazine nor phenytoin are effective in preventing barbiturate abstinence convulsions; a long-acting barbiturate in minimal effective doses permits smooth withdrawal in barbiturate addiction. (**Ref.** 1, p. 272; **Ref.** 6, pp. 353–354, 546–547; **Ref.** 8, pp. 535–538)

420. E. Short- to intermediate-acting barbiturates have been extensively used as hypnotics and have been shown in both sleep laboratories and clinical trials to be effective initially and over short-term periods for producing and maintaining sleep. (**Ref.** 1, p. 273; **Ref.** 3, p. 289; **Ref.** 6, pp. 86–87)

421. A. Although excessive chronic consumption of alcohol by an individual results in accumulation of fat and protein in the liver, which may proceed to cirrhosis, this is not part of the syndrome seen in the newborn. (**Ref.** 1, pp. 281–282; **Ref.** 6, pp. 375–376; **Ref.** 8, p. 373; **Ref.** 9, p. 539)

422. B. The benzodiazepines have a calming effect in doses much lower than those producing ataxia or measurable hypnosis. Their skeletal muscle relaxant effects are achieved through a central action, apparently in the reticular formation of the brain stem. They are effective in preventing seizure activity and in terminating ongoing convulsions. (**Ref.** 1, pp. 272–273; **Ref.** 2, p. 568; **Ref.** 4, p. 120; **Ref.** 8, pp. 350–352; **Ref.** 9, p. 441)

423. D. Temazepam is the second benzodiazepine approved for use as a hypnotic agent. Clinical studies indicated sleep and sleep maintenance parameters such as wake time after sleep onset, number of nocturnal awakenings, and residual medication effects were significantly improved by this drug. (**Ref.** 2, pp. 502–504; **Ref.** 3, p. 263; **Ref.** 9, pp. 444–445)

424. D. Cross tolerance exists to some degree to a wide range of CNS agents including sedative-hypnotics, narcotics, alcohol, and anesthetics. (**Ref.** 1, p. 272; **Ref.** 8, pp. 524–525; **Ref.** 9, p. 549)

425. A. Carbamazepine was first used to treat trigeminal neuralgia. It is not the first-line drug for the treatment of partial seizures. (**Ref.** 1, p. 292; **Ref.** 9, p. 491)

426. A. For absence seizures three drugs are available. They are ethosuximide, valproic acid, and clonezepam. Valoproic acid has an untoward effect of possible hepatotoxicity and it is difficult to establish the correct dosage of clonazepam. (**Ref.** 1, p. 300; **Ref.** 8, pp. 449–452, 458; **Ref.** 9, pp. 494–496)

427. D. Antiepileptic drugs act through various mechanisms, though all act partially or in full through reduction in the likelihood that the excessive discharges will spread over normal neurons. (**Ref.** 1, p. 289; **Ref.** 6, p. 449; **Ref.** 8, pp. 438–439)

428. A. Although it is questionable whether all children who have had seizure should receive any treatment, those at highest risk may profit by chronic therapy with phenobarbital. (**Ref.** 1, pp. 292–293; **Ref.** 6, p. 469; **Ref.** 8, pp. 445, 450)

429. E. Carbamazepine, like phenytoin, is effective in relieving generalized tonic-clonic seizures, but is ineffective in absence seizures and might make these seizures worse. (**Ref.** 1, pp. 291–292; **Ref.** 2, pp. 563–564; **Ref.** 3, p. 316; **Ref.** 8, pp. 449, 458; **Ref.** 9, p. 491)

430. D. Clonazepam is a benzodiazepine closely related to diazepam, but is more potent and is beginning to replace diazepam for use as an anticonvulsant. (**Ref.** 1, p. 298; **Ref.** 2, pp. 568–569; **Ref.** 3, p. 318; **Ref.** 8, p. 456; **Ref.** 9, p. 496)

431. C. Phenytoin, in adequate but minimal effective doses, usually does not cause sedation. (**Ref.** 1, pp. 288–289; **Ref.** 6, p. 450; **Ref.** 9, p. 489)

432. C. Colchicine also interferes with the deposition of urates in the joint by reducing the lactic acid content within the joint. (**Ref.** 1, p. 445; **Ref.** 6, p. 708; **Ref.** 8, pp. 674–675)

433. A. Aspirin, indomethacin, ibuprofen, and naproxen inhibit the synthesis of prostaglandins, which appears to be the mechanism responsible for their anti-inflammatory activity. (**Ref.** 1, pp. 436–438; **Ref.** 6, p. 674; **Ref.** 8, pp. 639–641; **Ref.** 9, p. 510)

434. D. Acetaminophen is more effective in treating minor pain and as an antipyretic. (**Ref.** 1, p. 444; **Ref.** 8, pp. 656–659; **Ref.** 9, pp. 514–515)

435. D. Hepatotoxicity may follow ingestion of a single dose of 10 to 15 g of acetaminophen; this toxic effect has been attributed to a metabolite that binds to cellular constituents, particularly glutathione. When production of the toxic metabolite exceeds the quantity of glutathione available for its inactivation, hepatotoxicity occurs. (**Ref.** 1, pp. 444–445; **Ref.** 4, p. 164; **Ref.** 6, p. 694; **Ref.** 8, pp. 658–659; **Ref.** 9, pp. 514–516)

436. B. Acetylcysteine (Muco-Myst) is a sulfhydryl compound which probably acts, in part, by replenishing hepatic stores of glutathione. Although its use for this purpose is considered experimental in the United States, it has been shown to be effective if given less than 24 hours after acetaminophen overdose. (**Ref.** 4, p. 164; **Ref.** 6, p. 694)

437. A. Although mefenamic acid has anti-inflammatory effects, its propensity for causing serious side effects limits its potential usefulness to short-term therapy. (**Ref.** 2, p. 591; **Ref.** 6, p. 698; **Ref.** 9, pp. 515–516)

438. E. Tolmetin, indomethacin, and sulindac constitute the acetic acid group of nonsteroidal anti-inflammatory drugs (NSAIDs). Tolmetin, in recommended doses, appears to be approximately equivalent in efficacy to moderate doses of aspirin, but is better tolerated. (**Ref.** 2, pp. 591–592; **Ref.** 6, p. 699; **Ref.** 8, pp. 663–664; **Ref.** 9, pp. 514–515)

439. C. Meclofenamate has been extensively used in laboratory animals as a prostaglandin synthetase inhibitor, and it is this property plus the ability to compete for binding at the prostaglandin receptor site which may be responsible for its anti-inflammatory actions. (**Ref.** 5, pp. 1541–1542; **Ref.** 6, pp. 698–699)

440. B. Diflunisal is a relatively new drug possessing significant anti-inflammatory but little antipyretic activity. It does not produce auditory side effects and appears to be less irritating to gastrointestinal mucosa. (**Ref.** 6, p. 689; **Ref.** 8, p. 669)

441. D. Probenecid is of no value in relieving pain and, in analgesic doses, aspirin is not uricosuric, but may actually block the effects of probenecid on uric acid excretion. (**Ref.** 3, p. 374; **Ref.** 8, p. 679)

442. C. The uricosuric actions of both aspirin and probenecid have been exploited for use in treatment of gout, with the latter being the more useful in the chronic or secondary form of the disease. (**Ref.** 1, pp. 445–446; **Ref.** 9, pp. 596–597)

443. A. Aspirin is suspected to increase the incidence of Reye's syndrome following cases of varicella and influenza. (**Ref.** 1, p. 435; **Ref.** 6, p. 683; **Ref.** 8, p. 647; **Ref.** 9, pp. 512–513)

444. A. In addition to the local irritation of the gastric mucosa, the damaging effect of aspirin may be due to inhibition of prostaglandins responsible for inhibition of gastric secretion in the intestines. (**Ref.** 6, p. 678; **Ref.** 8, pp. 651–652; **Ref.** 9, p. 511)

445. B. Probenecid is a weak acid related to benzoic acid and can slow the excretion of similar drugs. For example, it can alter the excretion of benylpenicillin and is used for that purpose. (**Ref.** 1, p. 838; **Ref.** 8, pp. 746, 1070–1073; **Ref.** 9, p. 596)

446. B. Salicylates inhibit the synthesis of prostaglandins in many areas including the peripheral tissues, thus interfering with sensitization of peripheral nerve endings to pain; they also reduce the irritability of the hypothalamus. (**Ref.** 2, p. 585; **Ref.** 3, pp. 367–368; **Ref.** 8, pp. 639–642; **Ref.** 9, pp. 510–511)

447. E. In addition, headache and lassitude will most likely be present. (**Ref.** 1, pp. 434–435; **Ref.** 6, pp. 491–495)

448. B. Toxic quantities of aspirin initially increase respiration, thereby reducing plasma CO_2, which results in renal excretion of sodium and potassium. Later, aspirin depresses respiration, allowing CO_2 to increase. The body does not contain sufficient sodium to prevent the development of respiratory acidosis. (**Ref.** 1, p. 755; **Ref.** 2, p. 558; **Ref.** 6, p. 682; **Ref.** 8, p. 646; **Ref.** 9, pp. 512–513)

449. E. There are at least 17 commonly used narcotic agents. These include morphine, codeine, fentanyl, and meperidine. The hypnotic-sedative diazepam, which is not a narcotic, is sometimes used in the place of narcotics in some situations. (**Ref.** 1, p. 372; **Ref.** 2, pp. 593–602; **Ref.** 8, pp. 490, 497)

450. B. All of these effects on the respiratory system make it advisable not to use morphine and related drugs during an asthmatic attack. Absorption from the gastrointestinal tract varies among drugs; meperidine, for example, being much more completely absorbed. (**Ref.** 1, pp. 374–375; **Ref.** 2, pp. 597–602; **Ref.** 6, p. 507; **Ref.** 8, p. 499)

451. E. Whereas the term opioid analgesics includes the products from opium and the somewhat chemically related narcotics, the term now includes the opiopeptins such as enkephalin. (**Ref.** 1, pp. 368–369; **Ref.** 2, pp. 593–608; **Ref.** 8, p. 486; **Ref.** 9, p. 518)

452. D. In the recumbent position, nausea after morphine administration is markedly less common; codeine shares with morphine the side effect of causing nausea and vomiting in some patients. (**Ref.** 1, p. 375; **Ref.** 2, pp. 597–599; **Ref.** 6, pp. 501–502; **Ref.** 8, p. 489; **Ref.** 9, p. 518)

453. D. More than 20 alkaloids have been identified as constituents of opium, but only three are important in therapeutics; ie, morphine, codeine, and papaverine. (**Ref.** 1, p. 368; **Ref.** 2, pp. 593–594; **Ref.** 6, pp. 491, 495; **Ref.** 9, p. 518)

454. E. Emesis, constipation, and respiratory depression are the common effects of the narcotics. Some patients experience euphoria. Myopia has to do with vision, miosis or pinpoint pupils is an effect of the narcotics. (**Ref.** 1, pp. 374–375; **Ref.** 2, pp. 597–580; **Ref.** 8, pp. 500–501; **Ref.** 9, pp. 521–522)

455. D. Although morphine reduces bile formation, the obstruction to its outflow elevates the bile pressure, causing distension of ducts within the liver (true for pancreatic juice and the pancreas also), and causing amylase and lipase to pass into the bloodstream. Atropine only partially relieves the spasm. (**Ref.** 1, pp. 374–376; **Ref.** 2, p. 598; **Ref.** 6, pp. 503–504; **Ref.** 8, pp. 495, 498–499; **Ref.** 9, p. 522)

456. E. The three findings—coma, pinpoint pupils, and depressed respiration—are known as the triad typical of acute opioid poisoning. Body temperature is reduced, resulting in a cold clammy skin. (**Ref.** 1, p. 374; **Ref.** 2, p. 597; **Ref.** 6, p. 509; **Ref.** 8, p. 500; **Ref.** 9, p. 523)

457. D. Morphine causes hyperglycemia indirectly by increasing catecholamine release from the adrenal, in turn causing glycogen in the liver to be converted to glucose. (**Ref.** 1, p. 374; **Ref.** 2, p. 579; **Ref.** 9, p. 522)

458. C. Although morphine and methadone are quite similar in many respects, methadone does differ in that absorption following oral administration is better and it stays in the organism longer. (**Ref.** 2, p. 572; **Ref.** 8, pp. 508–509)

459. B. Sudden withdrawal from an addictive drug is definitely inadvisable and may be life-threatening. Methadone substitution is one of the acceptable methods. (**Ref.** 1, pp. 384–385; **Ref.** 3, pp. 339–340; **Ref.** 8, pp. 560–561; **Ref.** 9, p. 547)

460. E. The intensity and duration of the symptoms are influenced by the degree of barbiturate dependence. Convulsions have occurred up to 7 days after withdrawal. (**Ref.** 1, pp. 385–386; **Ref.** 2, p. 588; **Ref.** 8, pp. 561–562; **Ref.** 9, p. 547)

461. D. Each precursor contains several biologically active opioids and nonopioid peptides that have been detected in blood and various tissues. (**Ref.** 1, p. 369; **Ref.** 6, pp. 492, 496)

462. B. Amphetamine has definite mood-elevating and analgesic effects, which enhance both euphoria and analgesia produced by the opioids. (**Ref.** 6, pp. 511, 525)

463. D. The respiratory depression produced by meperidine is equal to that seen with equianalgesic doses of morphine. This, along with the sedative effects, is rapidly antagonized by naloxone and other opioid antagonists. (**Ref.** 1, p. 379; **Ref.** 3, p. 328; **Ref.** 6, pp. 514–515, 526; **Ref.** 8, pp. 504–506; **Ref.** 9, p. 525)

464. C. One of the early uses of morphine and opium extracts was to treat diarrhea. Most morphine addicts suffer from chronic constipation. (**Ref.** 1, pp. 375–377; **Ref.** 2, pp. 597–602; **Ref.** 4, pp. 425, 1343–1344; **Ref.** 8, p. 504; **Ref.** 9, p. 523)

465. C. Naloxone is nearly a pure antagonist for morphine and the opioids. Given intravenously it will quickly overcome the depressant effects of the opioids. (**Ref.** 1, p. 381; **Ref.** 2, p. 603; **Ref.** 8, p. 516; **Ref.** 9, p. 527)

466. E. The eye responds to the drug with miosis. (**Ref.** 1, pp. 374–375; **Ref.** 2, pp. 597–602; **Ref.** 9, p. 523)

467. C. Morphine contains a complicated five-ring structure. (**Ref.** 1, pp. 373–376; **Ref.** 2, pp. 594–597; **Ref.** 8, pp. 489, 490; **Ref.** 9, p. 518)

468. A. Codeine is a methoxy-derivative of morphine that is produced by the opium plant. (**Ref.** 1, pp. 373–376; **Ref.** 2, pp. 594–597; **Ref.** 8, pp. 489, 490; **Ref.** 9, p. 518)

469. E. Naloxone is an opioid antagonist that contains a substitution on the *N*-group plus changes in the ring structure of the morphine molecule. (**Ref.** 1, p. 381; **Ref.** 2, p. 603; **Ref.** 8, pp. 489–490; **Ref.** 9, p. 527)

470. B. In contrast to pentylenetetrazol, in therapeutic doses methylphenidate is a mild CNS stimulant, but larger doses produce signs of generalized CNS stimulation which may lead to convulsions. (**Ref.** 1, pp. 101, 387; **Ref.** 6, pp. 585–586; **Ref.** 8, p. 213)

471. D. Although some analeptic drugs such as pentylenetetrazol have been used in an attempt to counteract severe CNS depression, this practice has been discredited by the success achieved by use of more conservative measures which stress intensive supportive care. (**Ref.** 6, p. 582)

472. B. Double-blind studies with placebo control have demonstrated that methylphenidate can improve both behavior and learning ability in 50% to 75% of these children, although indiscriminate use in such children is not approved. (**Ref.** 1, p. 427; **Ref.** 6, p. 587; **Ref.** 8, p. 427)

473. B. Methylphenidate is similar in action to amphetamine and has the same abuse potential. (**Ref.** 1, p. 387; **Ref.** 8, p. 213)

474. B. Caffeine is present in coffee and tea. Depending on how the coffee is made, a cup contains about 100 mg of caffeine. Patients are often warned about the use of coffee before certain medical procedures. (**Ref.** 3, p. 304; **Ref.** 8, p. 629)

475. A. Theophylline and aminophylline are used to treat asthma. The major side effects are nervousness and tremors. Increased doses can lead to restlessness, agitation, emesis, and tachycardia. (**Ref.** 1, p. 246; **Ref.** 8, p. 625)

476. A. Theophylline is the most effective bronchodilator of the natural xanthines. Aminophylline is a related xanthine that is effective in the treatment of asthma. (**Ref.** 2, p. 630; **Ref.** 3, p. 306; **Ref.** 8, p. 633)

477. A. Overdose of either drug may cause a range of symptoms of excessive CNS stimulation, but seizures are more likely to occur with theophylline; these seizures are occasionally refractory to anticonvulsant agents. (**Ref.** 6, p. 590; **Ref.** 8, p. 625)

478. B. All of these effects have been observed in individuals following the use of LSD, but the earliest and most persistent effect is mydriasis, which occurs even with very small doses. (**Ref.** 1, p. 388; **Ref.** 2, pp. 622–623; **Ref.** 6, pp. 564–565; **Ref.** 9, p. 553)

479. C. The prototype of the phenothiazine drugs, chlorpromazine, was developed as an antihistaminic, but was observed to have a beneficial effect in psychotic patients, thus leading to the introduction of a large number of related compounds for their antipsychotic activity. (**Ref.** 1, p. 359; **Ref.** 3, pp. 252–253; **Ref.** 6, pp. 391–392; **Ref.** 8, p. 386; **Ref.** 9, p. 462)

480. E. Amphetamines are known to release dopamine in the brain and can exacerbate schizophrenic symptoms, which are blocked by dopamine antagonists such as chlorpromazine. (**Ref.** 1, pp. 361–362; **Ref.** 2, pp. 536–538; **Ref.** 3, p. 247; **Ref.** 6, pp. 396–397; **Ref.** 8, p. 390; **Ref.** 9, p. 462)

481. D. The antipsychotic drugs are not used by addicts. They complain of how unpleasant the drugs make them feel. Antipsychotics produce a depressed feeling, urinary retention, and dry mouth. These agents cause hyperprolactinemia leading to amenorrhea, galactorrhea, and infertility. Occasionally extrapyramidal reactions interfere with therapy. (**Ref.** 1, pp. 351–352; **Ref.** 2, pp. 551–553; **Ref.** 9, p. 463)

482. C. The early antipsychotic drugs were derivatives of phenothiazine. The thioxanthene compounds are related to the phenothiazines. The butyrophenones, dihydroindolones, and dibenzoxazepines are not chemically related to the earlier antipsychotic drugs. (**Ref.** 1, p. 350; **Ref.** 2, p. 536; **Ref.** 3, pp. 253, 257–259; **Ref.** 8, p. 396; **Ref.** 9, p. 467)

483. E. The akathisia, impotence, psychoses, and tardive dyskinesia may occur with the antipsychotic agents. Tardive dyskinesia requires early detection because the condition may become permanent. (**Ref.** 1, p. 351; **Ref.** 2, p. 539; **Ref.** 8, p. 398; **Ref.** 9, p. 466)

484. C. The antipsychotics produce marked endocrine changes such as hyperprolactinemia. These effects include amenorrhea, galactorrhea, impotence, and decreased libido. (**Ref.** 1, p. 352; **Ref.** 2, pp. 537–539; **Ref.** 8, p. 392; **Ref.** 9, p. 464)

485. D. One of the first antidepressant agents, amintripyline, is still widely used. The second-generation agents include amoxapine, trazodone, maprotiline, and fluoxetine. (**Ref.** 1, p. 359; **Ref.** 2, p. 548; **Ref.** 3, p. 272; **Ref.** 8, pp. 405–407, 411)

486. C. The antidepressant drugs are divided into the tricyclic, second-generation tricyclic, and monoamine oxidase inhibitor agents. (**Ref.** 1, p. 359; **Ref.** 2, p. 548)

487. C. The prototype of the phenothiazine drugs, chlorpromazine, was developed as an antihistamine, but was observed to have a beneficial effect in psychotic patients, thus leading to the introduction of a large number of related compounds for their antipsychotic activity. (**Ref.** 3, pp. 251–256; **Ref.** 6, pp. 391–392; **Ref.** 8, pp. 391–392)

488. C. Trazodone was approved for use in 1982. The mechanism of its antidepressant action in humans is not fully understood, although it is not a monoamine oxidase inhibitor nor does it stimulate the CNS in the manner of amphetaminelike drugs. (**Ref. 1**, p. 360; **Ref. 2**, p. 556; **Ref. 5**, p. 1249; **Ref. 6**, p. 414; **Ref. 8**, p. 414; **Ref. 9**, p. 481)

489. A. Most of loxapine's effects on the CNS resemble those produced by the phenothiazines, although it appears less likely to cause sedation, weight gain, and extrapyramidal symptoms. (**Ref. 2**, p. 556; **Ref. 6**, pp. 393, 404; **Ref. 8**, p. 397; **Ref. 9**, p. 469)

490. D. Molindone produces moderate sedation, increased activity, and possibly euphoria without causing muscle relaxation or incoordination, apparently through an action on the reticular activating system. (**Ref. 2**, p. 556; **Ref. 5**, p. 921; **Ref. 6**, p. 504; **Ref. 8**, p. 397; **Ref. 9**, p. 470)

491. E. Haloperidol has less prominent tranquilizing properties than does chlorpromazine, although it shares the prominent side effect of production of extrapyramidal syndromes. Haloperidol is also useful in treatment of certain severe behavior problems in children. (**Ref. 2**, p. 501; **Ref. 3**, p. 260; **Ref. 6**, p. 405; **Ref. 8**, p. 397; **Ref. 9**, p. 468)

492. B. Amoxapine is of the same chemical class as loxapine, but is indicated for the relief of symptoms of depression in patients with certain neurotic and psychotic disorders, and thus is classified as an antidepressant rather than as an antipsychotic drug. (**Ref. 5**, p. 1088; **Ref. 6**, p. 413; **Ref. 9**, p. 468)

493. E. Haloperidol is a butyrophenone with the disadvantage of possible severe extrapyramidal syndrome. (**Ref. 1**, p. 350; **Ref. 8**, p. 397; **Ref. 9**, p. 468)

494. C. Thioridazine is an antipsychotic phenothiazine with a mild occurring extrapyramidal syndrome. (**Ref. 1**, p. 350; **Ref. 8**, p. 396; **Ref. 9**, p. 463)

495. D. Clozapine is a dibenzodiazepine antipsychotic drug with few side effects except for a reported 3% incidence of agranulocytosis. (**Ref. 1**, p. 350)

496. B. Amitriptyline is a prototype drug of the tricyclic class and it is a commonly used antidepressant with some sedative action. (**Ref.** 1, pp. 359–360)

497. A. The MAO inhibitors such as tranylcypromine, isocarboxazid, and phenylzine have been used to treat unusual depressions such as hypochondria and phobias. (**Ref.** 1, p. 264; **Ref.** 8, p. 417; **Ref.** 9, p. 494)

498. C. The toxic effects of imipramine include antimuscarinic effects and cardiac toxicity. (**Ref.** 2, pp. 550–552; **Ref.** 8, p. 405; **Ref.** 9, p. 478)

499. D. Potentiation of the effects of tricyclic drugs by methylphenidate can result from interference with their metabolism in the liver. (**Ref.** 2, pp. 554–555; **Ref.** 6, p. 422; **Ref.** 8, p. 405; **Ref.** 9, p. 478)

500. C. Imipramine and amitriptyline are the first of the tricyclic antidepressants. (**Ref.** 2, p. 550; **Ref.** 8, p. 405; **Ref.** 9, p. 478)

501. C. Although this and several other benzodiazepine compounds have skeletal muscle-relaxing properties, in controlled studies, they rarely show any advantage over either placebo or aspirin. (**Ref.** 3, p. 263; **Ref.** 6, p. 435)

502. A. The rapid onset of action of this drug is a consequence of its amphetaminelike action, and its sustained antidepressant effects are related to the inhibition of MAO. (**Ref.** 2, pp. 553–555; **Ref.** 8, p. 415)

503. D. It seems at present that chlorpromazine's hypotensive effect may be the result of an exaggeration of β-adrenergic vasodilation as it does not block the pressor action of norepinephrine. (**Ref.** 2, pp. 536–538; **Ref.** 3, p. 256)

504. A. The ingestion by patients on tranylcypromine of certain foods containing tyramine and other monoamines normally detoxified by MAO caused these severe hypertensive episodes. (**Ref.** 3, pp. 270–271; **Ref.** 8, p. 417; **Ref.** 9, p. 484)

505. B.   In contrast with single-dose administration, the phenothiazines, when given chronically, have adrenergic-potentiating
effects as reflected in potentiation of blood sugar responses to
norepinephrine. This potentiation is attributed to inhibition of the
catecholamine uptake mechanism, an action which readily occurs
peripherally, but not in the CNS. (**Ref.** 1, p. 347; **Ref.** 2, pp.
536–538)

506. A.   Chlorpromazine is effective in treating each of these
conditions, including nausea and vomiting induced by drugs and
by certain disease states, but it does not appear to control motion
sickness. (**Ref.** 1, p. 350; **Ref.** 2, p. 536; **Ref.** 3, p. 275; **Ref.** 6,
p. 411; **Ref.** 8, pp. 404, 927; **Ref.** 9, p. 465)

507. D.   The phenothiazine chlorpromazine as a rectal supposi-
tory is widely used as an antiemetic agent. It also produces sedation. (**Ref.** 1, p. 350; **Ref.** 6, pp. 411–412)

508. A.   Although phenothiazines do influence neuroendocrine
activity through depression of the hypothalamus, chlorpromazine
has been shown to stimulate rather than depress milk formation,
partly as a result of inhibition of prolactin release inhibiting hormone by the hypothalamus. (**Ref.** 1, p. 352; **Ref.** 2, pp. 539–540;
Ref. 6, p. 399; **Ref.** 8, p. 392)

509. A.   Extrapyramidal syndromes occur following the use of
almost all antipsychotic drugs, while agranulocytosis occurs only
rarely and is usually reversible if therapy is stopped immediately.
(**Ref.** 1, pp. 351–352; **Ref.** 2, pp. 539–540; **Ref.** 6, pp. 405–407;
Ref. 8, p. 398)

510. E.   A large number of drugs are known to possess antipsychotic properties, but because of poor clinical effectiveness or a
particular propensity for inducing side effects in required doses,
are not used for this purpose. (**Ref.** 1, p. 350; **Ref.** 5, p. 716; **Ref.** 6,
pp. 402, 412)

511. A.   The ability of certain drugs to produce antidepressant
effects without altering amine uptake and the lag between blockade of amine uptake and onset of antidepressant action by the

tricyclics have cast doubt on this as their mechanism of action. (**Ref.** 1, p. 349; **Ref.** 6, p. 416)

512. A. Lithium carbonate is given to replace sodium in the body. The lithium level of around 1 mEq/L in the serum is an average antipsychotic concentration. If this concentration is exceeded, tremors and mental confusion may occur. The lithium ion decreases thyroid function resulting in polydipsia and polyuria as the serum levels of lithium increase. (**Ref.** 1, pp. 355–359; **Ref.** 8, p. 418)

513. A. The EEG changes with the antipsychotic agents are first seen in the subcortical recording electrodes. It is possible that the underlying cause of the EEG changes may also induce occasional epileptic seizures in susceptible patients. (**Ref.** 1, p. 349; **Ref.** 8, p. 412)

514. A. The antipsychotic agents are powerful and are used to treat psychiatric conditions. Anxiety in the normal subject is better treated using the less depressing sedative-hypnotic drugs. (**Ref.** 1, pp. 351–352; **Ref.** 8, p. 403)

515. A. The antipsychotic drugs are not pleasant to take and there are major side effects. (**Ref.** 1, pp. 351–353)

516. C. One of the nonpsychotic uses of the phenothiazines is to prevent emesis especially following anesthesia and cancer chemotherapy. (**Ref.** 1, p. 350; **Ref.** 8, p. 927)

517. A. Lithium therapy involves replacing about 1 mEq/L of sodium in the serum. Somewhere above this concentration of lithium side effects are common. Therapy involves establishing a clinically effective dose of lithium and then maintaining that plateau level in the serum for a long time. Several things may alter this plateau including the increased renal clearance of lithium during pregnancy, the rebound after delivery, and the use of oral diuretics that produce a sodium loss. Sodium-induced loss reduces the amount of lithium that would be excreted. (**Ref.** 1, pp. 355–357)

7 Histamine, Serotonin, Prostaglandins, and Polypeptides

DIRECTIONS (Questions 518–531): Each of the questions or incomplete statements below is followed by five suggested answers or completions. Select the **one** that is best in each case.

518. Which of the following statements concerning angiotensin is false?
  A. Causes strong contractions of precapillary arterioles of skin, kidneys, and splanchnic area
  B. Increases the force of cardiac contractions, most likely by facilitating calcium entry as calcium channel blockers prevent this positive inotropic action
  C. Increases aldosterone secretion by the adrenals
  D. Has no direct action on the brain because the blood–brain barrier prevents its entry
  E. Increases vascular permeability, capillary filtration pressure, and extravascular fluid

519. When migraine is treated with ergotamine all of the following occur EXCEPT
  A. elevation of arterial pressure initially
  B. reduction of the carotid artery pulsation
  C. reduced hyperperfusion of area served by the basilar artery without modification of cerebral blood flow
  D. depression of the vasomotor center
  E. greater contraction of capacitance arteries than of small arterioles

520. Antihistamines (H_1) have varied clinical uses including
  A. decreased gastric secretion in peptic ulcer
  B. treatment of severe bronchial asthma attack
  C. increased blood flow to extremities in peripheral vascular disease
  D. treatment of cardiac arrhythmias
  E. prophylaxis and treatment of motion sickness induced by air, sea, or land travel

521. Antihistamines (H_1 antagonists) are useful in treating certain allergic disorders and the mechanism is most likely the result of
  A. inhibition of histamine release
  B. depletion of histamine stores
  C. metabolic inactivation of histamine following its release
  D. inhibition of histamine action by the antihistamine occupying histamine receptors
  E. chelation of histamine

522. Concerning serotonin antagonists, all of the following statements are true EXCEPT
  A. antagonism may involve several different mechanisms
  B. antagonism by cyproheptadine is an example of surmountable competitive type
  C. methysergide is of greatest benefit during migraine attacks
  D. antagonism of the effects of serotonin can be demonstrated with chlorpromazine and phenoxybenzamine
  E. antagonism can be achieved with numerous lysergic acid derivatives, many of which are naturally occurring ergot alkaloids

523. Histamine shock is associated with all of the following EXCEPT
   A. reduced venous return to the heart
   B. a decreased effective blood volume
   C. increased capillary permeability and edema
   D. engorged large blood vessels
   E. hemoconcentration

524. The H_2-receptor antagonists selectively block gastric acid secretion EXCEPT
   A. when stimulated by histamine
   B. when stimulated by gastrin
   C. from vagus nerve stimulation with electrical stimuli
   D. when caused by atropine
   E. nocturnal gastric secretions

525. Which of the statements concerning cyproheptadine is false?
   A. Side actions include dry mouth and drowsiness
   B. It reduces smooth muscle responses from carcinoid tumors
   C. It is effective in relieving the dumping syndrome which occurs after gastrectomy
   D. It is classified as an α-adrenergic antagonist
   E. Structurally it resembles the phenothiazine antihistamines

526. All of the following statements are true of histamine EXCEPT
   A. it is stored in mast cells and basophiles
   B. mast cells quickly restore the depletion of histamine
   C. it activates phosphatidyl inositol cycle
   D. it is a neurotransmitter
   E. it causes the "triple response"

527. Kinins are more potent than histamine on the vascular system and when injected intravenously produce all of the following effects EXCEPT
   A. brief fall in mean arterial blood pressure
   B. rapid fall in mean arterial blood pressure
   C. vasodilatation of blood vessels of the liver, kidney, heart, and skeletal muscle
   D. rapid dilation of the veins
   E. throbbing burning pain

528. Captopril (D-3 mercaptomethylpropanoyl-L-proline) is an inhibitor of converting enzyme in the renin-angiotensin system. Which of the following statements is true regarding captopril?
   A. Blocks the conversion of angiotensin I to angiotensin II
   B. Effective orally
   C. Used in the therapy of congestive heart failure
   D. Used in the treatment of hypertension
   E. All of the above

529. Renin secretion is inhibited by all of the following EXCEPT
   A. sodium ion
   B. potassium ion
   C. vasopressin
   D. angiotensin I
   E. angiotensin II

530. Angiotensin I acted upon by the converting enzyme, a dipeptidyl carboxypeptidase, yields angiotensin II. All of the following statements regarding angiotensin II are true EXCEPT
   A. increases the systolic and diastolic blood pressure
   B. acts on the central nervous system to induce drinking
   C. causes renal blood vessel dilatation
   D. stimulates aldosterone biosynthesis and release
   E. none of the above

531. Intravenously injected histamine in man exerts a variety of pharmacodynamic effects including those listed below EXCEPT
A. abrupt fall in the arterial blood pressure
B. an increase in heart rate
C. bronchoconstriction
D. increased gastric secretion
E. the "triple response"

DIRECTIONS (Questions 532–534): The group of questions below consists of five lettered headings followed by a list of numbered phrases or statements. For each numbered phrase or statement, select the **one** lettered heading that is most closely associated with it. Each lettered heading may be selected once, more than once, or not at all.

A. Cimetidine
B. Histamine
C. Bradykinin
D. Cyproheptadine
E. Diphenylhydantoin

532. Diagnostic aid in the determination of pernicious anemia

533. Antihistamine with potent antiserotonin activity

534. Effective in the treatment of the Zollinger-Ellison syndrome

---

DIRECTIONS (Questions 535–543): For each of the questions or incomplete statements below, **one** or **more** of the answers or completions given is correct. Select
A if only 1, 2, and 3 are correct
B if only 1 and 3 are correct
C if only 2 and 4 are correct
D if only 4 is correct
E if all are correct

Directions Summarized				
A	**B**	**C**	**D**	**E**
1,2,3	1,3	2,4	4	All are
only	only	only	only	correct

535. Which of the following statements is (are) true?
    1. About 90% of the serotonin in the body is located in the enterochromaffin of the intestines
    2. The brain contains only about 2% of the serotonin, though MAO inhibitors cause it to be twice that amount
    3. Massive carcinoid tumors may divert so much tryptophan to the synthesis of 5-hydrotryptamine, that pellagra may result
    4. The degradation product of serotonin is vanilly-mandelic acid (VMA), which is markedly increased by ingestion of bananas or treatment with reserpine

536. Effects of bradykinin include
    1. contraction of the rat uterus
    2. vasodilation, increased capillary permeability, and pain if injected (it should never be injected into tissues)
    3. bronchoconstriction in asthmatic patients
    4. bronchoconstriction in the guinea pig, which is blocked by aspirin

537. Which of the following statements is (are) correct concerning prostaglandins?
    1. Biosynthesis of prostaglandins starts from one of several 20-carbon essential fatty acids; in man linoleic acid and arachidonic acid are the most abundant precursors
    2. Prostaglandins are widely present in the body, in almost all tissues and body fluids, and act primarily at the site of their production
    3. Aspirin and nonsteroid anti-inflammatory drugs lower prostaglandin content of tissues and body fluids by inhibiting its synthesis
    4. Analogues of the fatty acid precursors of prostaglandins act as competitive inhibitors of the biosynthesis of prostaglandins

538. Which of the following statements is (are) true concerning prostaglandins (PG) E_2 and I_2?
1. They are potent antagonists to cholinergic-induced bronchoconstriction
2. They contribute to maintaining renal blood flow when cardiac output is low
3. They inhibit gastric acid and pepsin secretion
4. They cause relaxation of the nonpregnant uterus

539. Concerning the influence on platelet aggregation, which of the following statements is (are) true?
1. Prostaglandins D_2 and I_2 inhibit platelet aggregation by increasing the concentration of cyclic AMP
2. Prostacyclin is produced by the endothelium of blood vessels in minute amounts; 0.0003 parts per trillion inhibit aggregation
3. Thromboxane A_2, a metabolite of arachidonic acid, is a potent stimulator of platelet aggregation
4. Aspirin inhibits aggregation

540. Concerning captopril, which of the following statements is (are) correct?
1. If sodium depletion is present, it does not lower blood pressure
2. Administered orally, hypotension occurs within 20 minutes and continues for slightly more than 4 hours
3. It increases the effects of bradykinin and depresses aldosterone secretion
4. It does not modify the vascular response to administered angiotensin II or norepinephrine

541. The "triple response" produced by histamine given intradermally consists of
1. an early central red spot
2. a red flare of 1 or 2 cm in size appearing later
3. a white wheel replacing the original red spot
4. a long-lasting central red spot that gradually enlarges

Directions Summarized				
A	**B**	**C**	**D**	**E**
1,2,3	1,3	2,4	4	All are
only	only	only	only	correct

542. Vasoactive polypeptides include
    1. vasopressin
    2. substance P
    3. bradykinin
    4. serotonin

543. Untoward effects of H_2-receptor antagonists are
    1. constipation
    2. headache and dizziness
    3. vomiting
    4. a high incidence of blood dyscrasias

Explanatory Answers

518. D. Angiotensin does enter the brain, but in only a few areas. It can cause dipsosis and elevated sympathetic outflow from the brain. (**Ref.** 1, p. 219; **Ref.** 6, pp. 641–642; **Ref.** 8, p. 751)

519. A. Initially, ergotamine does not raise arterial pressure; however, a delayed, slow, moderate rise does occur and it causes a blockade of α-adrenergic endings and contraction of uterine muscles. (**Ref.** 1, pp. 211–214; **Ref.** 3, p. 229; **Ref.** 8, pp. 940, 942–944)

520. E. Cyclizine, promethazine, and meclizine (H_1 antagonists) are widely used in the prophylaxis of motion sickness. This action may relate to their anticholinergic and/or hypnotic effects. The best clinical results with H_1 antagonists are obtained in seasonal rhinitis, in which sneezing rhinorrhea and itching of the eyes, nose, and throat are relieved. (**Ref.** 1, p. 205; **Ref.** 2, p. 997; **Ref.** 3, pp. 218, 221; **Ref.** 6, p. 624; **Ref.** 8, p. 587; **Ref.** 9, p. 968)

521. D. The H_1 antagonists are the competitive type. However, they gain access to receptors only after the histamine on the receptors has been metabolized. (**Ref.** 1, pp. 203–204; **Ref.** 2, p. 997; **Ref.** 6, p. 623; **Ref.** 8, p. 581)

522. C. Methysergide, a potent serotonin antagonist, is useful only for the prevention and not for the treatment of migraine headaches. (**Ref.** 1, pp. 213–214; **Ref.** 3, p. 229; **Ref.** 6, p. 634; **Ref.** 8, p. 594)

523. D. Large blood vessels in histamine shock are collapsed and virtually emptied of blood, whereas the fine vessels are engorged. (**Ref.** 3, p. 203; **Ref.** 6, pp. 608–609; **Ref.** 8, pp. 607–608)

524. D. These tests are all used for the classification of the H_2-receptor antagonists. (**Ref.** 1, pp. 207–208; **Ref.** 8, pp. 899–900; **Ref.** 9, p. 961)

525. D. Cyproheptadine is classified as a serotonin-receptor antagonist. (**Ref.** 1, pp. 210–211; **Ref.** 8, p. 596)

526. B. Histamine is present in many cells of the body and the mast cells require approximately 2 weeks to restore their histamine content if it is depleted. (**Ref.** 1, pp. 200–203; **Ref.** 8, pp. 575–577; **Ref.** 9, pp. 961–962)

527. D. The kinins have a marked relaxing effect on the various arterial blood vessels of the bodily organs; however, the veins react with constriction. (**Ref.** 1, p. 222; **Ref.** 8, pp. 590–591; **Ref.** 9, p. 232)

528. E. Captopril and related converting enzyme inhibitors are easy to administer and are used to treat various cardiovascular diseases. (**Ref.** 1, p. 220; **Ref.** 8, p. 757; **Ref.** 9, p. 226)

529. D. Renin secretion is inhibited by a number of peptides and changes in serum potassium also alter secretion. Angiotensin I is nearly inactive on the biologic systems studied. (**Ref.** 1, p. 218; **Ref.** 8, p. 751; **Ref.** 9, p. 223)

530. E. While angiotensin I is nearly inactive, angiotensin II, which is a smaller peptide, is very active when injected into a local area such as the cerebral ventricle where it induces polydipsia. (**Ref.** 1, pp. 218–219; **Ref.** 8, p. 751; **Ref.** 9, p. 223)

531. E. The "triple response" is the result of intradermal injection of histamine. (**Ref.** 1, p. 200; **Ref.** 2, p. 995; **Ref.** 6, p. 607; **Ref.** 8, p. 580; **Ref.** 9, p. 962)

532. B. Histamine is useful as a diagnostic aid for differentiating pernicious anemia from other diseases of the stomach on the basis of achlorhydria. (**Ref.** 1, p. 203; **Ref.** 2, p. 996; **Ref.** 3, pp. 216–217; **Ref.** 6, p. 615; **Ref.** 8, p. 582; **Ref.** 9, p. 962)

533. D. Cyproheptadine is a potent inhibitor of histamine and serotonin, with some weak anticholinergic activity. It may be effective in postgastrectomy dumping syndrome. (**Ref.** 1, pp. 210–211; **Ref.** 3, pp. 223, 229; **Ref.** 6, p. 634; **Ref.** 8, p. 596; **Ref.** 9, p. 968)

534. A. Cimetidine causes a significant reduction in diurnal gastric acid secretion, reduces severity of peptic ulcers, and has been found to be effective in the treatment of the Zollinger-Ellison syndrome, which is due to slow-growing localized gastrin-secreting tumors in the pancreas and duodenum. (**Ref.** 1, pp. 207–208; **Ref.** 2, p. 1001; **Ref.** 3, p. 224; **Ref.** 6, p. 627; **Ref.** 8, p. 901; **Ref.** 9, p. 969)

535. A. The degradation product of serotonin is 5-hydroxyindoleacetic acid; VMA is the main degradation product of catecholamines. (**Ref.** 1, pp. 208–209; **Ref.** 3, pp. 108, 226–227; **Ref.** 8, p. 591)

536. E. Bradykinin may cause the release of prostaglandins. Bradykinin is a potent vasodilator; it increases capillary permeability, causes edema, and produces pain by acting on nerve endings. (**Ref.** 1, p. 221–222; **Ref.** 2, p. 267; **Ref.** 6, pp. 645–655; **Ref.** 8, p. 591)

537. A. Fatty acids in the diet such as phospholipids, triglycerides, and cholesterol esters serve as precursors for the synthesis of prostaglandins and thromboxanes. (**Ref.** 3, pp. 228–235)

538. E. Contractions of the gravid uterus are increased by PGE_2 as pregnancy progresses towards term. Any prostaglandins that may gain access to the blood are degraded in their first pass through the lungs, which prevents those from one organ from influencing tissues in another organ or another area. (**Ref.** 1, pp. 234–235; **Ref.** 3, pp. 228–235, 242; **Ref.** 6, p. 665; **Ref.** 8, p. 605; **Ref.** 9, p. 963)

539. E. By means of various products of arachidonic acid (PGs, TXs, HPETE, HETE, and the leukotrienes), the body either increases or decreases activities of tissues locally. (**Ref.** 1, pp. 229–234; **Ref.** 2, p. 384; **Ref.** 3, pp. 239, 242; **Ref.** 6, pp. 666, 668–669; **Ref.** 8, p. 603; **Ref.** 9, p. 561)

540. E. Captopril can cause a profound fall in blood pressure in malignant and renal hypertension. It can also lower blood pressure in other types of hypertension by the combination possibly of several mechanisms: i.e., interference with formation of angiotensin II, interference with the degradation of bradykinin, and depression of the secretion of aldosterone, thereby lowering tissue and plasma sodium concentrations. (**Ref.** 1, pp. 200–202; **Ref.** 3, p. 206; **Ref.** 6, pp. 649–651; **Ref.** 9, pp. 229–230)

541. A. The triple response results from intradermal injection of histamine and consists of (1) a central red spot (2) surrounded by a red flare of 1 to 2 cm, and (3) a white wheal replacing the original small red spot after about 2 minutes, due to edema. (**Ref.** 1, pp. 200–202; **Ref.** 2, pp. 921–924; **Ref.** 6, pp. 607–609; **Ref.** 8, p. 580; **Ref.** 9, p. 962)

542. A. Serotonin or 5-hydroxytryptamine is not a peptide. (**Ref.** 1, pp. 224–225; **Ref.** 8, p. 592; **Ref.** 9, p. 392)

543. A. The H_2-receptor antagonists are well-tolerated with only a small percentage of patients complaining of headache, dizziness, and sometimes constipation or vomiting. Cimetidine is associated with a few cases of blood dyscrasias making the condition rare considering the high volume usage of this drug. (**Ref.** 1, p. 208; **Ref.** 8, p. 899; **Ref.** 9, p. 969)

8 Drugs Affecting the Uterus and Locally Acting Gastrointestinal Drugs

DIRECTIONS (Questions 544–548): Each of the questions or incomplete statements below is followed by five suggested answers or completions. Select the **one** that is best in each case.

544. All of the following statements are true EXCEPT
   A. ergotamine, ergonovine, and bromocriptine are derivatives of lysergic acid
   B. caffeine increases the efficacy of ergotamine in relieving migraine
   C. ergot alkaloids cause contraction of muscles of the uterus and blood vessels and block α-adrenergic receptors
   D. prostaglandins act locally since they are destroyed in their first pass through the liver
   E. bromocriptine is a dopaminergic agonist, is effective in treating Parkinson's disease and acromegaly, and inhibits secretion of prolactin-secreting tumors

545. All of the following statements are true EXCEPT
  A. phenolphthalein stimulates the colon producing its effect in 6 to 8 hours; about 15% is absorbed and excreted mostly by the kidneys
  B. glycerin suppositories are useful, especially in children and older people, causing defecation usually in 30 minutes by its irritative hyperosmotic action on the rectal mucosa reflex
  C. magnesium-containing laxatives are the preferred laxatives for patients with severe renal damage
  D. psyllium hydrophilic mucolloid is a nonirritating bulk laxative
  E. kaolin, pectin, and bismuth subsalicylate are useful in treatment of diarrhea

546. The agent most likely capable of producing metabolic alkalosis is
  A. dioctyl sodium sulfosuccinate
  B. aluminum hydroxide
  C. magnesium trisilicate
  D. sodium bicarbonate
  E. calcium carbonate

547. All of the following statements are true EXCEPT
  A. ranitidine has a longer duration of action than cimetidine
  B. ergonovine is usually preferred over oxytocin to control postpartum bleeding because it causes more sustained uterine contractions
  C. antacids that elevate the pH above 4 but not above 5.5 do not tend to cause increased gastric acid secretion (acid rebound)
  D. ritodrine stimulates cholinergic receptors
  E. in metabolic acidosis, P_{CO_2}, HCO_3, and pH are initially decreased

548. All of the following statements are true EXCEPT
   A. oxytocin has very little stimulative action on the human uterus in the first trimester
   B. at term, infusion of very dilute oxytocin (1 μU/min initially, then after 30 minutes, slowly up to 4 μU/min) induces labor
   C. oxytocin causes and increases milk let-down in post-partum patients
   D. inhibition of prostaglandin (PG) synthesis reduces or abolishes uterine muscle response to oxytocin
   E. the aminopeptidase oxytocinase is produced by the placenta-degrading oxytocin but not vasopressin

---

DIRECTIONS (Questions 549–552): The group of questions below consists of five lettered headings followed by a list of numbered phrases or statements. For each numbered phrase or statement, select the **one** lettered heading that is most closely associated with it. Each lettered heading may be selected once, more than one, or not at all.

   A. Loperamide hydrochloride
   B. Ergonovine malleate
   C. Misoprostol
   D. Ritodrine
   E. Carboprost tromethamine

549. An analogue of PGE_1 and protects the gastric mucosa from acid and pepsin by increasing the secretion of mucus and by reducing other gastric secretions

550. Can act upon opiate receptors

551. An effective abortifacient as early as the 13th week of pregnancy

552. Use in individuals with insulin-dependent diabetes mellitus, cardiovascular problems, toxemia of pregnancy, or hyperthyroidism is dangerous and probably contraindicated

DIRECTIONS (Questions 553–555): For each of the questions or incomplete statements below, **one** or **more** of the answers or completions given is correct. Select

   A if only 1, 2 and 3 are correct
   B if only 1 and 3 are correct
   C if only 2 and 4 are correct
   D if only 4 is correct
   E if all are correct

553. Which of the following statements is (are) true?
 1. Pancreatic lipase convert castor oil to ricinoleic acid and glycerol. Ricinoleic acid stimulates peristalsis, moving material more rapidly through small and large intestines; the contents remain more fluid than usual
 2. All laxatives are contraindicated when abdominal pain is present; the cause has not been diagnosed
 3. Hiccups often can be eliminated by chlorpromazine or by inhalation of carbon dioxide with oxygen added
 4. Many physicians suggest that households with children should have syrup of Ipecac available in their medicine cabinets

554. Which of the following statements is (are) true?
 1. Cimetidine penetrates the blood–brain barrier less than ranitidine
 2. Sucralfate is a combination of sucrose and aluminum which combines with proteins and this compound forms a protective coat to the ulcer
 3. Omeprazole stops premature labor by inhibiting synthesis of prostaglandins in the uterus
 4. Oxytocin produces relaxation of arterial smooth muscle including those of the coronary arteries

555. Which of the following statements is (are) true?
1. Since gastric lavage is contraindicated in a comatose poisoned patient, an intramuscular injection of an emetic is preferred
2. Dioctyl sodium sulfosuccinate is a detergent and softens the stools by keeping water in the feces
3. If a physiologic antagonist exists for the mechanism poisoned, its use is indicated in most cases of poisoning
4. Chlorpromazine and promethazine are phenothiazines that are useful in the treatment of nausea and vomiting

Explanatory Answers

544. D. The lungs are the only organs that receive all of the venous blood in their capillary vessels and is the site of first pass destruction of prostaglandins, thereby restricting them to local sites of action. The lungs also remove other substances including the kinins, some catecholamines, and serotonin. (**Ref. 3**, pp. 218–219, 305, 516; **Ref. 8**, pp. 473, 942, 943)

545. C. About one third of orally administered magnesium may be absorbed and this is normally excreted by the kidneys; however, in individuals with severe renal damage severe magnesium toxicity may occur. (**Ref. 3**, pp. 523–526; **Ref. 4**, p. 743; **Ref. 8**, pp. 705, 916–917, 920–921)

546. D. Sodium bicarbonate is a systemic antacid and can cause metabolic alkalosis with no proportional increase in Pco_2. (**Ref. 3**, p. 520; **Ref. 4**, 743)

547. D. Ritodrine stimulates β_2-adrenergic receptors, thereby inhibiting uterine contractions. It is one of several adrenergic agonists that can prevent premature labor. (**Ref. 3**, pp. 212, 577–578; **Ref. 8**, pp. 693, 943, 949–950)

548. E. Oxytocinase degrades both oxytocin and vasopressin. At term and during labor prostaglandin levels in maternal blood, fetal blood, and amniotic fluid are elevated. During the last two trimesters of pregnancy labor begins after the administration of PGE_2 or PGF_2. (**Ref. 3**, p. 577; **Ref. 8**, pp. 937, 938, 948)

549. C. Misoprostol is useful in preventing ulcers in patients taking aspirin over prolonged periods of time. It is effective in healing gastric, but not duodenal, ulcers. It should not be given when conception might occur as it is an abortifacient. (**Ref. 8**, pp. 610–611; **Ref. 9**, p. 987)

550. A. Loperamide is an effective antidiarrheal agent; structurally it is related to haloperidol and acts upon opiate receptors. (**Ref. 3**, pp. 340–341, 523; **Ref. 8**, p. 925; **Ref. 9**, p. 976)

551. E. Carboprost tromethamine is the methyl derivative of prostaglandin F and is injected intramuscularly. Dinoprostone, 20 mg suppositories, are inserted into the vagina. Both preparations are abortifacients and may cause side effects of nausea, vomiting, diarrhea, and fever. (**Ref.** 3, p. 578; **Ref.** 8, p. 938; **Ref.** 9, p. 567)

552. D. When insulin-dependent diabetes mellitus patients receive ritodrine, insulin should be given to prevent ketoacidosis. (**Ref.** 8, p. 950)

553. E. Syrup of Ipecac in a dose of 15 mL, followed by some water, can be expected to produce emesis in about 30 minutes. (**Ref.** 8, pp. 57, 341, 404, 922, 923; **Ref.** 9, pp. 980–981)

554. C. Cimetidine penetrates the blood–brain barrier more readily than ranitidine. Omeprazole strongly inhibits the gastric acid pump and is especially useful in reducing acid secretion in Zollinger-Ellison syndrome. (**Ref.** 4, pp. 743–744; **Ref.** 8, pp. 903–904, 910, 936)

555. C. In comatose poisoned patients, gastric lavage is preferred over emetics because there is less danger of aspiration of the material and because most emetics depress the central nervous system. (**Ref.** 8, pp. 59–60, 922, 927–928; **Ref.** 9, pp. 980–981)

9 Chemotherapy

DIRECTIONS (Questions 556–565): Each of the questions or incomplete statements below is followed by five suggested answers or completions. Select the **one** that is best in each case.

556. Syphilis in a patient allergic to penicillin G would be treated with
    A. amoxicillin
    B. ampicillin
    C. erythromycin
    D. amphotericin B
    E. biltricide

557. The effectiveness of penicillin can be increased by simultaneous administration of probenicid which acts to
    A. decrease protein binding of penicillin
    B. decrease glomerular filtration of penicillin
    C. decrease renal tubular reabsorption of penicillin
    D. decrease renal tubular secretory transport of penicillin
    E. increase renal tubular reabsorption of penicillin

558. The tendency to become drug resistant during treatment is highly developed in the etiologic agent of tuberculosis. This problem is usually avoided by
  A. increasing the dose when resistance develops
  B. simultaneous probenicid administration
  C. combined therapy with isoniazid and another drug such as rifampin
  D. simultaneous use of three sulfonamides
  E. restriction of fluid intake

559. The preference for benzathine penicillin in primary syphilis depends on
  A. reduced number of doses required
  B. higher peak drug levels in the blood
  C. fast dispersion from injection site
  D. absence of allergic potential
  E. oral dosage possibility

560. In some systemic infections due to invasive fungi, amphotericin B is usually given with
  A. sulfadiazine
  B. ampicillin
  C. dactinomycin
  D. flucytosine
  E. tolnaftate

561. The most serious adverse effect of penicillin is
  A. hearing loss in the high-frequency range
  B. anaphylaxis due to allergy
  C. renal failure
  D. hepatitis
  E. metabolic and nutritional disturbances

562. Chancroid caused by *Hemophils ducreyi* is best treated with
  A. trimethoprim and sulfamethoxazole
  B. sulfadiazine
  C. tetracycline
  D. penicillin G
  E. streptomycin

563. Acetylation refers to the
  A. mechanism of action of sulfonamides
  B. recommended doses of sulfonamides
  C. metabolic inactivation of sulfonamides
  D. diffusion of sulfonamides in the body
  E. bacteriostatic effect of sulfonamides

564. The most common toxic side effect due to isoniazid therapy is
  A. peripheral neuritis
  B. hypersensitivity
  C. optic neuritis
  D. dryness of the mouth
  E. convulsion

565. A folic acid antagonist useful as an antineoplastic and immunosuppressive drug is
  A. cyclophosphamide
  B. azathioprine
  C. doxorubicin
  D. methotrexate
  E. procarbazine

DIRECTIONS (Questions 566–573): Each group of questions below consists of a diagram with five lettered components, followed by a list of numbered phrases or statements. For each numbered phrase or statement, select the **one** lettered component that is most closely associated with it. Each lettered component may be selected once, more than once, or not at all.

Questions 566–569 (Figure 11):

566. Antibacterially inactive product formed by the action of penicillinase or gastric acid on the penicillin molecule

567. Substitution on the penicillin molecule at this site may result in alteration of susceptibility of the resultant compounds to inactivating enzymes and may change the antibacterial activity and pharmacologic properties of the drug

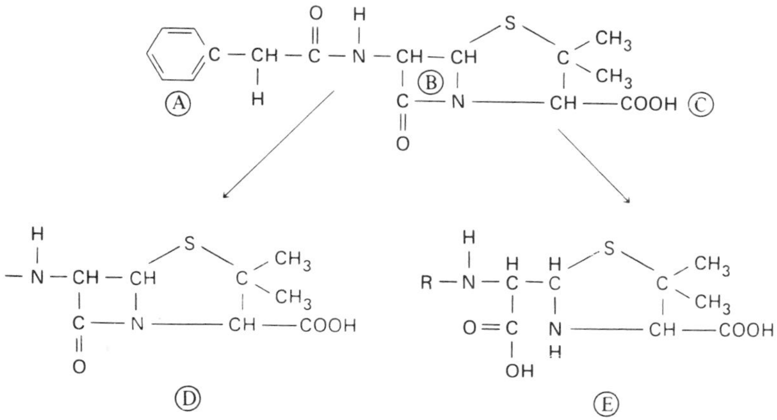

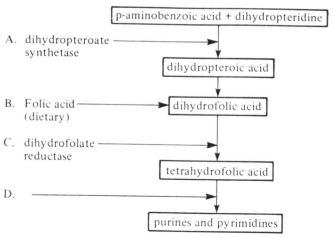

Figure 11

568. The presence of this moiety in the compound identifies it as penicillin G

569. The basic structure of all the penicillins, which can be obtained by the action of bacterial amidases on penicillin

Questions 570–573 (Figure 12):

Figure 12 Folic acid in metabolism.

570. This step occurs in humans and may occur in some bacteria

571. Sulfamethoxazole exerts its antimicrobial effect by competing at this site in the bacterial life cycle

572. Antibacterial site of action of trimethoprim

573. Although selective toxicity of the trimethoprim-sulfamethoxazole combination on bacterial cells is achieved in two ways, the metabolic consequences of the two actions are indicated in this step

DIRECTIONS (Questions 574–610): Each group of questions below consists of lettered headings followed by a list of numbered words, phrases, or statements. For each numbered word, phrase, or statement select the **one** lettered heading that is most closely associated with it. Each lettered heading may be selected once, more than once, or not at all.

Questions 574–577:

    A. Carbenicillin
    B. Cefamandole
    C. Chloramphenicol
    D. Erythromycin
    E. Piperazine

574. Recommended for treatment of Legionnaire's disease.

575. Dicarboxylic acid which is useful in serious infections caused by *Pseudomonas* spp.

576. Has been fatal to infants due to their inability to conjugate the drug with glucuronic acid and excrete it

577. Nonpenicillin β-lactam antibiotic which is active against most gram-positive cocci, *Hemophilus influenzae*, *Aerobacter aerogenes*, *Klebsiella* spp., and *Proteus* spp.

Questions 578–582:

- **A.** Metronidazole (Flagyl)
- **B.** Emetine hydrochloride
- **C.** Paromomycin (Humatin)
- **D.** Praziquantel (Biltricide)
- **E.** Thiabendazole (Mintezole)

578. Poorly absorbed drug suitable for asymptomatic carriers of *Entamoeba histolytica*

579. Cardiotoxic alkaloid effective in amebic dysentery

580. Rapidly absorbed drug effective in all forms of schistosomiasis in three oral doses in one day

581. Drug effective in oral administration in strongyloidiasis and recommended in trichinosis

582. Synthetic heterocyclic drug effective in large doses against both intestinal and extraintestinal infection with *Entamoeba histolytica*

Questions 583–587:

- **A.** Oxamniquine
- **B.** Mebendazole
- **C.** Pyrimethamine and sulfadiazine
- **D.** Niclosamide
- **E.** Diethylcarbamazine

583. Effective against whipworm (trichuriasis) and ascariasis

584. An alternative drug for *Schistosoma mansoni* infection

585. Effective against *Toxoplasma gondii*

586. Effective against filariasis due to *Wuchereria bancrofti* in an 18-day course

587. Effective in tapeworm infections due to beef, pork, and fish tapeworms

Questions 588–592:

    A. Pyrantel pamoate
    B. Praziquantel
    C. Diiodoquin
    D. Niridazole
    E. Chloroquine

588. Drug of choice for dwarf tapeworm infection

589. Effective against guinea worm infection (*Dracunculus medinensis*) and alternative in schistosomiasis

590. Alternative drug in hepatic infection with *Entamoeba histolytica*

591. Alternative to mebendazole in pinworm infection

592. A poorly absorbed alternative for mild diarrhea due to *Entamoeba histolytica*

Questions 593–597:

    A. Doxorubicin
    B. Streptomycin
    C. Penicillin G
    D. Dactinomycin
    E. Azaribine

593. Antimetabolite useful in psoriasis

594. Inhibits cocci and gram-positive rod-shaped bacteria but not tubercle bacilli

595. Causes myocardial degeneration

596. Useful in methotrexate-resistant choriocarcinoma

597. Lethal to sensory cells of inner ear

Questions 598–601:

    A. Mechlorethamine
    B. Oncovin
    C. Procarbazine
    D. Prednisone

598. The most rapidly acting alkylating agent

599. Derivative of methylhydrazine, a weak monoamine oxidase inhibitor and potentiator of alcohol toxicity in addition to cytotoxic action

600. A meticorticoid which has selective toxicity for lymphocytes

601. An alkaloid of the periwinkle plant which with prednisone produces 90% remission rate in acute lymphoblastic leukemia in children

Questions 602–605: ABVD stands for adriamycin, bleomycin, vinblastine, and dacarbazine.

    A. Adriamycin
    B. Bleomycin
    C. Vinblastine
    D. Dacarbazine

602. A glycopeptide antibiotic produced by *Streptomyces*, with activity against carcinomas of various sites as well as Hodgkin's disease and with less bone marrow toxicity than most cancer chemotherapy drugs

603. Tetracycline glycoside antibiotic that binds DNA, especially cardiac DNA

604. A linear triazine which is cleaved in cells to an alkylating agent and an intermediate of inosine metabolism

605. Mitosis inhibitor due to affinity for the protein tubulin, a constituent of microtubules

Questions 606–610:

    A. Potassium iodide
    B. Miconazole
    C. Mefloquine
    D. Ketoconazole
    E. Griseofulvin

606. Useful against blastomycosis, histoplasmosis, coccidiomycosis, and candidiasis but not against fungal meningitis

607. Useful against infections of the skin, hair, and nails caused by species of *Microsporum, Trichophyton,* and *Epidermophyton*

608. Produces a high rate of cure of vaginal candidiasis, mycotic infections of the feet and groin, as well as tinea versicolor by topical administration

609. Effective against lymphocutaneous sporotrichosis

610. Effective against *Plasmodium vivax* and *Plasmodium falciparum*

DIRECTIONS (Questions 611–619): Each set of lettered headings below is followed by a list of numbered words or phrases. For each numbered word or phrase select

    A if the item is associated with **A** only
    B if the item is associated with **B** only
    C if the item is associated with both **A** and **B**
    D if the item is associated with neither **A** nor **B**

Questions 611–614:

    A. Cefoperazone
    B. Ceftriaxone
    C. Both
    D. Neither

611. Effective against typhoid fever

612. A large fraction of the dose is excreted in the bile

613. Half-life of elimination exceeds 5 hours

614. First choice in all forms of gonorrhea unless the local strains are known to be sensitive to penicillin

Questions 615–617:

    A. Cefoxitin
    B. Metronidazole
    C. Both
    D. Neither

615. Important in treatment of *Endameba histolytica* infection

616. Active against gram-negative anaerobic infections, eg, infections with *Bacteroides fragilis*

617. Classified as β-lactam antibiotics

Questions 618 and 619:

    A. Cefoperazone
    B. Ceftazidime
    C. Both
    D. Neither

618. Shows strong activity against *Pseudomonas aeruginosa*

619. Oral administration is the usual method

DIRECTIONS (Questions 620–650): For each of the questions or incomplete statements below, **one** or **more** of the answers or completions is correct. Select

A if only 1, 2, and 3 are correct
B if only 1 and 3 are correct
C if only 2 and 4 are correct
D if only 4 is correct
E if all are correct

620. Vancomycin possesses which of the following useful properties?
   1. Effective against methicillin-resistant staphylococci
   2. A glycopeptide available as the soluble hydrochloride salt
   3. Synergistic with gentamicin against *Staphylococcus aureus* and *Streptococcus faecalis*
   4. Can be used in patients who are allergic to penicillin

621. Polymyxins have which of the following characteristics?
   1. They are peptide antibiotics
   2. They are cationic detergents
   3. They alter permeability of bacterial cell membranes
   4. They are only administered parenterally

622. The tetracyclines have which of the following characteristics?
   1. After parenteral administration, they are excreted in the feces as well as the urine
   2. They are usually given by oral administration but intravenous and intramuscular forms are available
   3. They cause a dose-dependent gastrointestinal irritation which is reduced by the presence of food
   4. They bind 30S subunits of ribosomes and block transfer of amino acids from t-RNA

623. Which of the following statements is (are) correct with regard to clindamycin?
   1. Available as the hydrochloride salt for oral use and the phosphate salt for parenteral administration
   2. Penetrates the central nervous system with ease
   3. Effective against *Bacteroides fragilis*
   4. The drug of first choice against enterococci

624. The synergistic combination of trimethoprim and sulfamethoxazole (Bactrim or Septra) has which of the following useful characteristics?
   1. Inhibits two steps in bacterial synthesis of tetrahydrofolic acid
   2. Reduces the likelihood of development of drug-resistant strains of bacteria
   3. Effective against *Pneumocystis* and *Nocardia*
   4. Effective in chronic infections of the urinary tract

625. Zidovudine (3′-azido-3′-deoxythymidine or AZT)
   1. causes decreased short-term mortality in patients with acquired immunodeficiency syndrome (AIDS)
   2. is converted in vivo to a triphosphate nucleotide which is a competitive inhibitor of reverse transcriptase of HTLV-III
   3. is effective by oral administration
   4. increases the frequency and severity of opportunistic infections of patients with AIDS

626. Idoxuridine causes
   1. altered transcription of the base sequence of herpes viral DNA
   2. synthesis of abnormal viral DNA
   3. inhibition of herpes viral replication
   4. inhibition of reverse transcriptase of herpes virus

627. Characteristics of cyclosporine include
   1. ability to inhibit rejection of organ transplants
   2. inhibition of isomerases that control conformational folding of proteins
   3. inhibition of lymphokine production by helper T cells
   4. severely myelosuppressive in therapeutic doses

		Directions Summarized		
A	**B**	**C**	**D**	**E**
1,2,3	1,3	2,4	4	All are
only	only	only	only	correct

628. Prophylactic use of antibiotics in surgery is not necessary in many operations, but in certain kinds of operations antibiotics are given to reduce the risk of infection. These include
   1. gastrointestinal surgery with impaired motility and impaired acid production
   2. appendectomy when the appendix is gangrenous
   3. surgery of the head and neck when the oral and pharyngeal mucosa is penetrated
   4. urinary tract surgery in subject with nonsterile urine

629. Which of the following statements regarding the action of drugs against malaria is (are) true?
   1. Chloroquine-resistant strains are most likely *Plasmodium falciparum*
   2. Relapses of malaria due to *Plasmodium vivax* can be cured with primaquine plus chloroquine
   3. Mefloquine is used to treat strains resistant to chloroquine
   4. *Plasmodium falciparum* gametocytes are more sensitive to primaquine than to chloroquine

630. Drugs used with dapsone against leprosy to avoid drug resistance include
   1. mycelex
   2. rifampin
   3. flucytosine
   4. clofamazine

631. Carmustine, lomustine, and semustine are nitrosoureas containing a chlorethyl group and are correctly described as
   1. semisynthetic antibiotics
   2. used in Hodgkin's disease
   3. useful in tuberculosis and leprosy
   4. alkylating agents

632. Which of the following drugs are used in AIDS, not for their antiviral effect, but for their effect on opportunistic infection?
   1. Pentamidine
   2. Trimethoprim
   3. Sulfamethoxazole
   4. Zidovudine

633. An accurate characterization of amantadine would include
   1. curative for influenzas A, B, and C
   2. prophylactic for influenza A
   3. active against DNA viruses but not RNA viruses
   4. inhibits the uncoating process which initiates the viral growth cycle in the host cell

634. Tests in lymphocyte cultures infected with HTLV-III have revealed antiviral activity at low concentrations in which of the following substances?
   1. D-penicillamine
   2. Avarol, which is obtained from the sponge *Dysidea avara* and avarone, a quinone obtained from the oxidation of avarol
   3. Amphotericin B methyl ester
   4. Phosphonoformate (Foscarnet)

635. Which of the following are characteristics of interferons?
   1. Proteins
   2. Produced in response to virus and other types of infection
   3. Inhibitory for a wide variety of unrelated viruses
   4. Nontoxic parenterally and nonirritating when used topically on the nasal mucosa

636. Synthetic inducers of interferon production include
   1. double-stranded RNA polymers
   2. pyran (polymer of divinyl ether and maleic anhydride)
   3. tilerone
   4. prednisone

		Directions Summarized		
A	**B**	**C**	**D**	**E**
1,2,3	1,3	2,4	4	All are
only	only	only	only	correct

637. Encouraging clinical results with interferon have been observed in
    1. bladder cancer, breast cancer, malignant melanoma, cancer of the head and neck, osteogenic sarcoma, and cervical cancer when it is used as an adjunct to surgery
    2. malaria
    3. acute fulminant hepatitis, spreading herpes simplex in immunosuppressed patients, and viral encephalitis
    4. osteoarthritis

638. Which of the following fungi are not inhibited by flucytosine?
    1. *Cryptococcus neoformans*
    2. *Histoplasma capsulatum*
    3. *Candida albicans*
    4. *Blastomyces dermatitidis*

639. Flucytosine can be correctly described as
    1. an alkaloid
    2. a pyrimidine base analogue
    3. an antibiotic
    4. an antimetabolite

640. Which of the following statements is (are) correct concerning nifurtimox?
    1. Trypanosomicidal for *Trypanosoma cruzi*
    2. Curative in acute or chronic Chaga's disease
    3. Effective by oral administration
    4. Causes toxic effects on the central nervous system

641. Selection of an antimicrobial agent should take into account
1. the causative organism
2. the tendency to develop drug resistance
3. whether the patient can tolerate the toxic effects of treatment
4. absorption and distribution of the drug which determine the route of administration

642. The type of drug resistance that is transferred during bacterial conjugation depends on
1. bacteriophage
2. selection of inducible enzyme
3. selection of random genetic mutations
4. two DNA factors

643. The transpeptidation reaction, which forms a peptide bond between adjacent strands of peptide glycan polymer, is inhibited by
1. cephalothin
2. tetracycline
3. penicillin
4. streptomycin

644. The action of bacitracin on bacterial cell wall synthesis involves inhibition of
1. dephosphorylation of the phospholipid carrier
2. messenger-RNA synthesis
3. folic acid synthetase
4. D-alanyl-D-alanine synthetase

645. Which of the following drugs are bone marrow depressants?
1. Dactinomycin
2. Daunorubicin
3. Fluorouracil
4. Mercaptopurine

Directions Summarized				
A	**B**	**C**	**D**	**E**
1,2,3	1,3	2,4	4	All are
only	only	only	only	correct

646. Chronic lymphocytic leukemia is initially treated with an alkylating agent such as
   1. prednisone
   2. cytosine arabinoside
   3. 6-thioguanine
   4. chlorambucil

647. In chronic granulocytic leukemia hydroxyurea has certain advantages over busulfan. These are
   1. less risk of severe myelosuppression
   2. does not require allopurinol
   3. less chronic pulmonary toxicity
   4. broad spectrum of activity

648. In acute nonlymphocytic leukemia in children treatment may result in severe infections which can be treated with
   1. cephalothin, gentamicin, and carbenicillin
   2. amphotericin B
   3. trimethoprim and sulfamethoxazole
   4. prednisone and praziquantel

649. Acute myelogenic leukemia in adults can be put in remission with
   1. amantadine and ribavirin
   2. allopurinol and sulfadiazine
   3. dapsone and clofazamine
   4. cytosine arabinoside and daunorubicin

650. Which of the following are "rescue" techniques to protect normal cells from lethal damage by certain antimetabolites used as antineoplastic agents?
  1. Administration of leucovorin (folinic acid, citrovorum factor) with folate analogues
  2. Administration of thymidine with folate analogues
  3. Administration of leucovorin and thymidine with folate analogues
  4. Administration of leucovorin and thymidine with purine or pyrimidine analogues

Explanatory Answers

556. C. Amoxicillin and ampicillin may cause anaphylactic shock or other allergic reactions in subjects allergic to penicillin G. The antimicrobial spectrum of erythromycin is penicillinlike and includes *Treponema pallidum*. (**Ref.** 4, p. 242; **Ref.** 8, p. 1134)

557. D. Probenicid also inhibits renal tubular secretion of methotrexate and biliary secretion of rifampin. Probenicid is unusual in that its half-life of elimination is dependent on dose. (**Ref.** 3, p. 646; **Ref.** 8, pp. 746, 1073)

558. C. The choice of drugs for tuberculosis should be based on in vitro tests of the causative organism isolated from the patient and should include isoniazid, if possible. (**Ref.** 3, p. 672; **Ref.** 8, p. 1146)

559. A. Benzathine penicillin is a sparingly soluble salt which is slowly dispersed from an intramuscular injection site, producing bactericidal plasma concentration for 2 weeks. (**Ref.** 3, p. 648; **Ref.** 8, pp. 1070, 1071)

560. D. Advantages of flucytosine are: effectiveness of oral administration, penetration into the cerebrospinal fluid, and less toxicity compared with amphotericin B. The combination with amphotericin B is preferred in order to avoid the emergence of strains resistant to flucytosine. (**Ref.** 3, p. 680; **Ref.** 8, pp. 1174, 1175)

561. B. Anaphylaxis due to penicillin is a life-threatening reaction involving severe hypotension or bronchoconstriction. It may involve angioedema, nausea, and vomiting. The incidence is approximately one in a thousand treated subjects. (**Ref.** 3, p. 648; **Ref.** 8, p. 1081)

562. A. Resistance to sulfonamide alone or tetracycline is likely to be a problem. The toxicity of streptomycin is a serious problem. The synergistic pair of sulfamethoxazole and trimethoprim is recommended. (**Ref.** 4, p. 246; **Ref.** 8, p. 1057)

563. C. The major metabolic derivative is N^4-acetyl-sulfonamide, which retains the toxic potentialities but not the therapeutic properties of the parent compound. (**Ref.** 1, p. 1109; **Ref.** 8, p. 1049)

564. A. Peripheral neuritis, which occurs in 2% of patients receiving 5 mg/kg of isoniazid daily, can be prevented by concurrent administration of pyridoxine. (**Ref.** 1, p. 1202; **Ref.** 8, p. 1148)

565. D. Methotrexate induces remissions in leukemia, is effective in choriocarcinoma, and is useful as an immunosuppressive agent in organ transplants. (**Ref.** 1, p. 1272; **Ref.** 3, p. 702; **Ref.** 5, pp. 762–764; **Ref.** 8, p. 1226)

566. E. Gastric acid and β-lactamases, such as penicillinase, hydrolytically open the β-lactam ring to form penicilloic acid, which is devoid of antibacterial activity. (**Ref.** 2, pp. 625–626; **Ref.** 4, p. 427)

567. A. Resistance to destruction by gastric acid, resistance to bacterial penicillinase, and the spectrum of antibacterial activity are all determined to a large extent by the nature of the moiety attached to the amino group of 6-amino-penicillanic acid. (**Ref.** 3, pp. 642, 643; **Ref.** 8, pp. 1065–1066, 1076)

568. A. Benzylpenicillin is penicillin G, the first useful antibiotic discovered, the only natural penicillin used clinically, and still the most important and widely used antibiotic. (**Ref.** 8, pp. 1065, 1076)

569. D. 6-Amino-penicillanic acid, a molecule which contains a double-ring structure consisting of a β-lactam ring and a thiazolidine ring, and by itself possessing significant antibacterial activity against some gram-negative organisms, is the major structural requirement for penicillin activity. (**Ref.** 8, p. 1064)

570. B. Humans do not synthesize folic acid and many lower organisms cannot use preformed folates. (**Ref.** 8, pp. 1048, 1054)

571. A. Sulfonamides are structural analogues of para-aminobenzoic acid (PABA) and thus prevent bacterial utilization of PABA; specifically they inhibit dihydropteroate synthetase, the enzyme responsible for incorporation of PABA into dihydropteroic acid, the immediate precursor of folic acid. (**Ref.** 3, p. 634; **Ref.** 8, p. 1054)

572. C. The action of trimethoprim on the enzyme dihydrofolate reductase gives this compound a toxic potential on cells that utilize preformed folic acid as well as those that synthesize it. (**Ref.** 8, p. 1054)

573. D. Tetrahydrofolic acid, acting as a carrier of methylene groups, participates in the synthesis of purines by supplying carbon atoms numbered 2, 4, and 5 of the purine ring and participates in the synthesis of deoxythymidylic acid by supplying the methyl group added to position number 5 by thymidylate synthetase. When these reactions are blocked in bacteria, reproduction is inhibited by the failure of DNA and RNA synthesis. (**Ref.** 8, pp. 1054, 1302; **Ref.** 17, pp. 729, 739)

574. D. Erythromycin is effective against *Legionella* spp. associated with pneumonia and endocarditis. Combination therapy with rifampin is recommended. (**Ref.** 8, p. 1133; **Ref.** 18, p. 176)

575. A. Carbenicillin is administered parenterally in large doses against gram-negative infections which are not much affected by penicillin G or ampicillin. Attention needs to be given to the large amount of sodium given in the doses required. (**Ref.** 3, p. 651; **Ref.** 8, pp. 1080–1081)

576. C. The drug-metabolizing systems of the liver and the excretory function of the kidney are not fully developed at birth. Fatal toxicity may result if these facts are not taken into account in the dose. (**Ref.** 8, p. 1129)

577. B. Cefamandole represents a broadened spectrum of activity obtained by variations in structure of groups attached to the 7-amino-cephalosporanic acid nucleus, which is characteristic of the cephalosporins. (**Ref.** 8, pp. 1086, 1089)

578. C. Paromomycin is an aminoglycoside antibiotic. Diloxanide furoate is also suitable for asymptomatic carriers. (**Ref.** 8, pp. 1000–1001, 1005)

579. B. Emetine hydrochloride is so toxic that patients taking it should be in the hospital but it is also extremely toxic to amebae and quickly controls severe amebic dysentery. (**Ref.** 8, p. 1001)

580. D. Praziquantel is rapidly metabolized and excreted, mostly as metabolites, in the urine. It causes stimulation followed by spastic paralysis in schistosomes. Side effects are abdominal discomfort, headaches, and dizziness. (**Ref.** 3, pp. 698, 700; **Ref.** 8, p. 479)

581. E. Thiabendazole is effective against a variety of nematode infections of humans and animals. It is believed to be beneficial in the early intestinal stage of trichinosis and in cutaneous larva migrans. (**Ref.** 2, pp. 621–622; **Ref.** 8, pp. 957, 970, 971, 972)

582. A. The asymptomatic carrier state of *Entamoeba histolytica* infection is not always terminated by metronidazole. This drug is also useful against *Trichomonas vaginalis* infection and *Giardia lamblia* infection. (**Ref.** 2, p. 694; **Ref.** 8, pp. 1002–1005)

583. A. Mebendazole is also used against hookworm infection of both kinds and is active against guinea worm and *Loa loa*. It has an affinity for intracellular microtubules of worms. (**Ref.** 8, pp. 963–964)

584. A. Oxamniquine is a nitroquinoline that has a highly specific toxicity for *Schistosoma mansoni*, particularly the males. In Brazil it is given in a single oral dose. (**Ref.** 3, pp. 698, 701; **Ref.** 8, p. 966)

585. C. These drugs are synergistic in their action against toxoplasmosis. Leucovorin (folinic acid) should be given concurrently to protect against bone marrow suppression. (**Ref.** 8, pp. 987, 1009, 1053)

586. E. Diethylcarbamoyl-*N*-methyl piperazine effectively removes the microfilariae making the blood noninfective for mosquitoes. Higher doses are believed to kill adult worms. (**Ref.** 3, pp. 698, 700; **Ref.** 8, p. 973)

587. D. Although niclosamide is effective in killing *Taenia solium*, the eggs are not killed. If the dead worms are not promptly removed, the eggs may give rise to cysticercosis. For this reason praziquantel may be preferable for pork tapeworm infection. (**Ref.** 3, pp. 698, 700; **Ref.** 8, pp. 957, 960–961)

588. B. Niclosamide is also very effective. (**Ref.** 8, p. 957)

589. D. Niridazole is more effective against *Schistosoma haematobium* than *Schistosoma mansoni*. In the 5- to 10-day course of oral treatment it causes considerable toxicity including central nervous system effects. Praziquantel is preferred in schistosomiasis and metronidazole in guinea worm infection. (**Ref.** 3, pp. 698, 701; **Ref.** 8, pp. 956, 958, 965)

590. E. Because of the high concentrations it reaches in the liver and its considerable amebicidal activity, chloroquine is a suitable substitute for metronidazole in hepatic amebiasis. (**Ref.** 8, p. 1001; **Ref.** 18, p. 38)

591. A. Pyrantel pamoate is a poorly absorbed, relatively safe, highly effective drug for ascaris, pinworm, and both kinds of hookworm. (**Ref.** 3, pp. 698, 699; **Ref.** 8, pp. 969–970)

592. C. A drug used for decades against intestinal amebiasis. Diiodoquin may cause optic atrophy. Diloxanide furoate may be a safer choice. (**Ref.** 3, pp. 688, 689; **Ref.** 8, p. 1001)

593. E. This acetylated derivative of azauridine has been associated with intravascular clotting and emboli. Azauridine is an analogue of cytosine arabinoside, which is an important drug for acute myelocytic leukemia. (**Ref.** 8, pp. 1188, 1189, 1228, 1232)

594. C. It is worth noting that penicillin G is bactericidal to gram-negative as well as gram-positive cocci and also to spirochetes. Acquired resistance in staphylococci is overcome with methicillin or oxacillin and resistance in gonococci by ceftrioxone. (**Ref.** 8, pp. 1069, 1075–1078, 1090)

595. A. Positive results with a wide range of cancers have stimulated a search for less toxic analogues of doxorubicin. Epirubicin and idarubicin are products of this effort. (**Ref.** 2, p. 774; **Ref.** 8, pp. 1206, 1241)

596. D. This chromopeptide antibiotic from *Streptomyces* is given in 5-day courses by the intravenous route in doses denominated in micrograms per kilogram body weight. In combination with vincristine and other measures, dactinomycin is curative in Wilm's tumor. (**Ref.** 2, p. 778; **Ref.** 8, p. 1240)

597. B. Streptomycin, the prototypical aminoglycoside antibiotic, shares with gentamicin and tobramycin a specific toxicity for the hair cells of the cochlea. Degeneration is progressive beginning in the cells responding to high-frequency sounds. (**Ref.** 2, p. 651; **Ref.** 8, pp. 1104–1105)

598. A. Two combinations of four drugs each have been much used to treat Hodgkin's disease. The combination of mechlorethamine, oncovin, procarbazine, and prednisone is called MOPP. The other effective combination (ABVD) consists of adriamycin, bleomycin, vinblastine, and dacarbazine. Mechlorethamine, the first alkylating agent used in cancer chemotherapy, is given intravenously; care must be taken so that the drug does not come into contact with subcutaneous tissues. (**Ref.** 2, p. 759; **Ref.** 3, p. 703; **Ref.** 8, pp. 1215–1216)

599. C. Procarbazine is absorbed after oral administration, albeit incompletely. It is metabolized to mutagenic compounds which cause acute leukemia in some subjects. It is also immunosuppressive. (**Ref.** 2, p. 785; **Ref.** 3, pp. 704, 710; **Ref.** 8, p. 1252–1253)

600. D. Modification of the structure of hydrocortisone yields meticorticoids, which show a toxicity to lymphoid tissues and have proven to be useful against lymphoid neoplasia. (**Ref.** 2, p. 820; **Ref.** 8, pp. 1253–1254, 1442, 1457)

601. B. The vinca alkaloids, vincristine and vinblastine, bind to microtubules and produce a disorder of mitosis in which cell division is halted in metaphase. Vincristine shows less bone marrow suppression than vinblastine. (**Ref.** 2, p. 780; **Ref.** 3, p. 709; **Ref.** 8, pp. 1236–1239)

602. B. Bleomycin binds DNA and causes chromosome breaks. It may cause ulceration of the skin and fibrosis of the lungs. Together with vinblastine and cisplatin, it is curative in testicular carcinoma. (**Ref.** 2, pp. 755, 775; **Ref.** 3, p. 709; **Ref.** 8, pp. 1244–1246)

603. A. Adriamycin is a synonym for doxorubicin. ABVD is used in Hodgkin's disease and lymphoma. Doxorubicin is also used in the induction of remissions in acute lymphocytic leukemia in adults (with vincristine and prednisone). (**Ref.** 8, pp. 1241–1243; **Ref.** 18, p. 345)

604. D. Dacarbazine is metabolized to an alkylating agent which is active against malignant melanoma. (**Ref.** 2, p. 767; **Ref.** 8, pp. 1222–1223)

605. C. Vinblastine is active against testicular cancer in combination with bleomycin and cisplatin. (**Ref.** 2, p. 781; **Ref.** 8, p. 1238)

606. D. Ketoconazole is recommended over amphotericin B in patients who are not gravely ill. It may cause gynecomastia and sterility in men and menstrual disorders in women owing to reduction of steroid synthesis. It may also cause hepatitis. (**Ref.** 2, p. 734; **Ref.** 3, p. 679; **Ref.** 8, pp. 1171–1174)

607. E. Griseofulvin given orally is deposited in skin, hair, and nails where it prevents infection of newly formed cells. Duration of therapy depends on the time required for complete replacement of infected tissue. Many toxic effects are described. (**Ref.** 2, p. 731; **Ref.** 3, pp. 679, 681; **Ref.** 8, pp. 1173, 1174)

608. B. Miconazole has a slightly higher cure rate for dermatophytosis than tolnaftate (Tinactin). (**Ref.** 2, p. 734; **Ref.** 3, pp. 679, 680; **Ref.** 8, p. 1171)

609. A. A saturated solution of potassium iodide is diluted and given orally. Hypersensitivity to iodine may be encountered. Amphotericin B is required in other forms of sporotrichosis. (**Ref.** 2, p. 734; **Ref.** 8, p. 1175)

610. C. Mefloquine is a synthetic fluorinated analogue of quinine, which suppresses *Plasmodium vivax* malaria and produces cure of *P. falciparum* malaria including many drug-resistant strains. (**Ref.** 8, pp. 987–988)

611. C. Both of these third-generation cephalosporins may be preferable to chloramphenicol, which causes agranulocytosis and aplastic anemia in rare instances. (**Ref.** 2, p. 658; **Ref.** 3, p. 661; **Ref.** 8, pp. 1092, 1127)

612. C. As with chloramphenicol and ampicillin, significant concentrations of drugs appear in the bile. The combination of trimethoprim and sulfamethoxazole is also effective in typhoid fever and both components are excreted in bile as well as urine. (**Ref.** 8, pp. 1055, 1090)

613. B. Ceftrioxone has a half-life of 8 hours, the longest among currently available cephalosporins. The half-life of cefaperazone is 2.1 hours. (**Ref.** 8, p. 1090)

614. B. Ceftriaxone is the first choice in all forms of gonorrhea unless local strains are known to be sensitive to penicillin. (**Ref.** 8, pp. 1090–1091)

615. B. Metronidazole is effective in both intestinal and extraintestinal amebiasis in a course of orally administered treatment lasting 10 days. (**Ref.** 3, p. 687; **Ref.** 8, p. 1003)

616. C. Other possible choices are cefotetan and clindamycin. (**Ref.** 8, pp. 1089, 1137)

617. A. Cefoxitin is a cephamycin, a subgroup of β-lactam antibiotics closely related to cephalosporins. Metronidazole is hydroxyethylmethyl-nitro-imidazole. (**Ref.** 8, pp. 1002, 1085–1086)

618. C. Other cephalosporins may show useful activity against gram-negative bacteria but fail against *Pseudomonas*. Other β-lactams that are effective are carbenicillin, ticarcillin, azlocillin, mezlocillin, and pipercillin. (**Ref. 8**, pp. 1080–1081, 1088–1090)

619. D. The oral β-lactam antibiotics are penicillin V, ampicillin, oxacillin, cloxacillin, dicloxacillin, amoxicillin, carbenicillin-indanyl, cephalexin, cephradine, cefadroxal, and cefaclor. (**Ref. 8**, pp. 1076–1077, 1086–1087)

620. E. Vancomycin is bactericidal to various gram-positive bacteria including staphylococci and streptococci. In toxicity it resembles aminoglycosides: ototoxicity and nephrotoxicity. It inhibits cell wall synthesis of bacteria. (**Ref. 2**, p. 665; **Ref. 3**, p. 654; **Ref. 8**, pp. 1138–1140)

621. B. Polymyxin B is useful in mixtures for topical application to surface injuries that are in danger of becoming contaminated. Combined with bacitracin and neomycin it forms a mixture with a broad spectrum of activity. (**Ref. 2**, p. 666; **Ref. 8**, pp. 1138, 1584)

622. E. The tetracyclines inhibit bacterial protein synthesis by blocking the addition of amino acids to the growing polypeptide. Streptomycin and other aminoglycosides also bind to the 30S subunit where they block the initiation of protein synthesis or cause errors of transcription of the RNA template. (**Ref. 2**, p. 653; **Ref. 3**, pp. 630, 659; **Ref. 8**, pp. 1100, 1118)

623. B. Like erythromycin and chloramphenicol, clindamycin inhibits protein synthesis in susceptible bacteria by binding to 50S ribosomes. (**Ref. 2**, p. 660; **Ref. 3**, p. 662; **Ref. 8**, pp. 1134–1137)

624. E. The components have similar half-lives of elimination which helps to maintain an approximately constant ratio of drugs after oral administration. Attention should be given to maintaining adequate urinary volume. (**Ref. 2**, pp. 611, 618; **Ref. 8**, p. 1055)

625. A. This analogue of thymidine causes granulocytopenia and anemia in many patients. (**Ref. 8**, pp. 1182–1184; **Ref. 10**, p. 8333; **Ref. 15**, pp. 185, 190)

626. A. In the form of ophthalmic ointments and solutions, idoxuridine is useful against herpes simplex keratitis especially when the infection is confined to the epithelium. (**Ref.** 2, p. 687; **Ref.** 3, p. 667; **Ref.** 8, p. 1188; **Ref.** 11, p. 111)

627. D. In contrast to methotrexate and azathioprine, cyclosporine does not cause bone marrow suppression. It causes renal, hepatic, and nervous system toxicity. (**Ref.** 3, pp. 724, 725; **Ref.** 8, pp. 1267, 1268)

628. E. Surgery in uncontaminated sites does not require prophylactic antibiotics. When surgery is done in contaminated sites, an antibiotic should be selected on the basis of the microorganisms most likely to be present. (**Ref.** 8, p. 1042; **Ref.** 12, pp. 105–108)

629. E. Chloroquine phosphate, in a single dose once each week, has been widely used for malaria prophylaxis in travelers. In areas where chloroquine-resistant *Plasmodium falciparum* is found, it is important to consider other choices. (**Ref.** 3, p. 692; **Ref.** 8, p. 983)

630. C. Rifampin is a broad-spectrum, semisynthetic antibiotic which inhibits bacterial RNA polymerase. Resistance develops readily and the causative agent of leprosy is prone to become resistant to drugs, hence the need for multiple-drug treatment. (**Ref.** 3, p. 675; **Ref.** 8, p. 1160)

631. C. Carmustine and lomustine cross the blood–brain barrier, an important property in therapy of leukemia. All three drugs are bone marrow suppressants. (**Ref.** 2, pp. 763, 764; **Ref.** 8, pp. 1220–1222)

632. A. Pentamidine and the combination of trimethoprim and sulfamethoxazole are active against *Pneumocystis*, an important pathogen in immunodeficient subjects. (**Ref.** 8, p. 1012; **Ref.** 16, p. 375)

633. C. Amantadine is a readily absorbed, persistent (half-life, 16 hours) tricyclic amine which prevents influenza A when given before symptoms appear and ameliorates the illness when given early in the development of symptoms. (**Ref.** 2, p. 685; **Ref.** 3, p. 667; **Ref.** 8, pp. 1191–1192)

634. E. Phosphonoformate has been used experimentally in subjects with AIDS to treat cytomegalovirus infections and herpes simplex type 2 infections. (**Ref.** 8, p. 1189; **Ref.** 13, pp. 416, 417, 419)

635. A. Interferons are rapidly removed from the plasma after parenteral administration and are irritants when used topically to prevent virus infections of the nasal mucosa. (**Ref.** 8, pp. 1189–1190; **Ref.** 14, pp. 456, 460, 461, 494–497)

636. A. Synthetic RNA polymers are not suitable inducers for clinical use because of their toxicity, which resembles the toxicity of interferon: fever, leukopenia, nausea, and abnormalities of liver and bone marrow. (**Ref.** 14, pp. 461, 462)

637. B. There is at present a great interest in the use of interferons in cancer and virus diseases owing to the availability of interferon from recombinant DNA technology. (**Ref.** 8, pp. 1189–1191; **Ref.** 14, pp. 487–494)

638. C. *Histoplasma capsulatum* and *Blastomyces* are inhibited by amphotericin B. (**Ref.** 8, p. 1166)

639. C. Flucytosine is 5-fluorocytosine and is therefore a pyrimidine base analogue. It can act as an antimetabolite in two ways, by being converted to 5-fluorouridylic acid, or to 5-fluorodeoxyuridylic acid which is an inhibitor of thymidylate synthetase. (**Ref.** 2, p. 732; **Ref.** 3, p. 680; **Ref.** 8, p. 1168)

640. E. The treatment is by oral administration and is continued for 90 to 120 days. Numerous toxic effects include nervous system effects. In some areas, chronic infections do not respond. (**Ref.** 3, pp. 691, 696; **Ref.** 8, pp. 1010–1011)

641. E. Other important factors may be age, pregnancy, drug interaction, drug allergy, and the half-life of elimination which determines the frequency of administration. (**Ref.** 2, pp. 603–612; **Ref.** 8, pp. 1022–1037)

642. D. The gram-negative enterobacteria such as *E. coli* and *Salmonella* species exchange genes through a temporary intercellular bridge. A resistance determinant plasmid and a resistance transfer factor (RTF) must be transferred to induce resistance in progeny of a previously sensitive cell. (**Ref.** 3, p. 628; **Ref.** 8, pp. 1021–1022)

643. A. The cell wall of staphylococci is a polymer of *N*-acetylglucosamine chains cross-linked by amino acid chains. In the final step of polymerization a molecule of alanine is displaced from one chain while its adjacent amino acid (also alanine) is bonded to the terminal glycine of another chain. The formation of this alanine–glycine bond is the step inhibited by β-lactam antibiotics. (**Ref.** 17, pp. 762–764)

644. D. The dipeptide of D-alanine is synthesized and then added to a peptide side chain which will form a cross-link of the peptidoglycan. The synthesis of the dipeptide is inhibited by bacitracin. Vancomycin inhibits the bonding of the dipeptide to L-lysine. (**Ref.** 17, pp. 762–764)

645. E. With few exceptions antineoplastic drugs are potent and nonspecific inhibitors of cell multiplication. (**Ref.** 2, p. 751; **Ref.** 8, pp. 1204, 1214, 1221, 1223, 1225, 1227, 1230, 1236, 1237, 1243)

646. D. Chlorambucil is given orally at the highest tolerated dose for as long as the disease is stable or asymptomatic. (**Ref.** 8, p. 1219; **Ref.** 8, p. 367; **Ref.** 16, p. 379)

647. B. Busulfan is associated with pulmonary fibrosis. Both drugs require allopurinol to prevent uric acid toxicity. (**Ref.** 8, p. 1220; **Ref.** 18, p. 362)

648. A. Trimethoprim and sulfamethoxazole prevent *Pneumocystis* pneumonia. Ceftazidime is an alternative for bacterial infections. Amphotericin B is added if fever persists. (**Ref.** 18, p. 361)

649. D. Allopurinol is needed to prevent uric acid nephropathy. Both drugs cause neutropenia and thrombocytopenia. (**Ref.** 18, p. 355)

650. A. The term "rescue" has been applied to techniques that utilize leucovorin and/or thymidine to protect normal tissues from lethal damage by folic acid analogues such as methotrexate, thus allowing the use of higher doses effective against certain tumors that otherwise would not be responsive. (**Ref.** 2, p. 768; **Ref.** 8, p. 1224)

10 Toxicology

DIRECTIONS (Questions 651–660): Each of the questions or incomplete statements below is followed by five suggested answers or completions. Select the **one** that is best in each case.

---

651. Concerning cyanide (hydrocyanic acid, prussic acid), all of the following statements are correct EXCEPT
    A. cyanide is one of the most rapidly acting poisons
    B. cyanide had a very high affinity for iron in the ferric state, reacting readily with the trivalent iron of cytochrome oxidase in mitochondria; cellular respiration is thus inhibited and cytotoxic hypoxia results
    C. diagnosis of cyanide poisoning may be facilitated by the characteristic odor of bitter almonds on the breath of the victim, an odor with which the physician should be familiar
    D. treatment of cyanide poisoning consists of nitrite by inhalation and intravenously, and sodium thiosulfate to convert hemoglobin to methemoglobin, which has great affinity for cyanide ion and removes it from binding to cytochrome oxidase
    E. acute toxicity is not likely to result from ingestion of cyanide because of its incomplete absorption from the gastrointestinal tract

652. The CNS effects experienced by those engaging in the drug-abuse phenomenon of "glue sniffing" are due to the action of the solvent
    A. isopropanol
    B. benzene
    C. propylene glycol
    D. toluene
    E. diethylene glycol

653. Concerning carbon monoxide, all of the following statements are correct EXCEPT
    A. carboxyhemoglobin is a compound that dissociates most rapidly in the presence of pure oxygen, which displaces carbon monoxide in the hemoglobin molecule and converts carboxyhemoglobin to oxyhemoglobin
    B. although the formation of carboxyhemoglobin decreases the oxygen-carrying capacity of the blood, it does not decrease the Po_2 of arterial blood and as a result there is no stimulation of chemoreceptors
    C. anemic persons are more susceptible to carbon monoxide poisoning than are individuals with normal amounts of hemoglobin
    D. the toxic reactions that result from exposure to carbon monoxide are primarily the result of tissue hypoxia produced by the inability of the blood to transport sufficient oxygen
    E. when exposed to a given concentration of carbon monoxide, children succumb later than do adults

654. Concerning organic solvents, all of the following statements are correct EXCEPT
   A. inhalation of high concentrations of gasoline vapors in confined quarters may result in sudden death
   B. inhalation of kerosene vapor is less hazardous than is the ingestion of kerosene
   C. gasoline vapors, like other hydrocarbons, may cause sensitization of the myocardium to catecholamines and ventricular fibrillation, and/or rapid CNS depression and respiratory failure
   D. ethanol is useful in the treatment of methanol poisoning
   E. hypotension associated with carbon tetrachloride poisoning is best treated by the intravenous administration of norepinephrine

655. All of the following statements are true of lead poisoning EXCEPT
   A. it may be either acute or chronic, but acute poisoning occurs relatively infrequently
   B. of the three chelating agents most commonly employed in its treatment, only penicillamine is effective when given orally
   C. organic lead compounds are more likely to produce CNS symptoms, while aberrations in hemoglobin synthesis are more apt to be associated with inorganic lead poisoning
   D. exposure to lead occasionally produces unmistakable, progressive mental deterioration in children
   E. lead poisoning constitutes a lesser hazard in children since the lead is more rapidly deposited in developing bones, thus diverting it from tissues of potential toxicity

656. With regard to mercury poisoning, all of the following statements are true EXCEPT

    A. three major forms of the metal must be distinguished: mercury vapor (elemental mercury), salts of mercury, and organic mercurials

    B. the primary tissue target of chronic toxicity of elemental mercury vapor is the kidney

    C. mercury has a special affinity for the sulfur atom in thiol groups of enzymes to inactivate them, which is ultimately responsible for its toxicity

    D. mercury may be absorbed via the respiratory and gastrointestinal tracts as well as the skin

    E. the upper limit of a normal concentration of mercury in blood is 0.01 to 0.03 μg/mL

657. All of the following statements are true of arsenic EXCEPT

    A. both inorganic forms of arsenic are readily available, mainly in industrial products and in some medicines

    B. the pathways and products of biotransformation of arsenic have not been well-defined

    C. dimercaprol is the primary agent used in the treatment of chronic arsenic poisoning

    D. arsenic readily crosses the blood–brain barrier

    E. arsenic produces dilatation of capillaries and an increase in permeability of the capillary walls

658. Organophosphorus insecticides such as diazinan, dichlorvous, and parathion inhibit cholinesterases. All of the following are reported acute toxic effects EXCEPT

    A. salivation

    B. miosis

    C. sweating

    D. bronchial dilatation

    E. vomiting

659. Polychlorinated biphenyls (PCBs) were used in electrical transformers, in many articles as plasticizers, and flame retardants, etc, until 1977. The PCBs are stable and lipid soluble and are found in our foods. Workers exposed to high concentrations of PCBs developed which of the following reactions:
    A. stomach ulcers
    B. chloracne, rash, hyperkeratosis
    C. low sperm count
    D. acute pulmonary edema
    E. diarrhea

660. Treatment of acute carbon monoxide poisoning should include all of the following EXCEPT
    A. hyperbaric oxygen (where available)
    B. maintenance of respiration
    C. immediate notification of next of kin
    D. removal from exposure source
    E. administration of oxygen

661. All of the following effects are evidence of arsenic toxicity EXCEPT
    A. blood, casts, and protein in urine
    B. vesicles under the intestinal mucosa
    C. polycythemia
    D. peripheral neuropathy
    E. facial edema

DIRECTIONS (Questions 662–663): The group of questions below consists of five lettered headings followed by a list of numbered statements. For each numbered statement, select the **one** lettered heading that is most closely associated with it. Each lettered heading may be selected once, more than once, or not at all.

Questions 662–663: Chelators used as metal antidotes form stable bonds with the metals. This combination, metal–chelator, is nonpolar and is excreted by the kidney. The metals below are treated with one of the chelators below.

A. Mercury
B. Copper
C. Iron
D. Zinc
E. Tin

662. Deferoxamine is antidote for which metal above

663. Dimercaprol is the antidote for which metal above

Explanatory Answers

651. E. Cyanide gas is highly toxic when inhaled, as demonstrated by its use for executions in so-called gas chambers; its highly lethal properties when taken by mouth have also been brought to public attention recently by its use in more than 900 religious "suicide-murders" in Guyana and by its substitution for medication in capsules on drugstore shelves in the "Tylenol murders" in the United States. (**Ref.** 3, p. 729; **Ref.** 6, pp. 1642–1643; **Ref.** 8, pp. 1630–1631)

652. D. Commercial toluene is the solvent for glue; however, it contains other hydrocarbons including benzene. The mental confusion from the mixture is greater than additive. (**Ref.** 1, p. 737; **Ref.** 3, pp. 733–734; **Ref.** 6, pp. 1637–1638; **Ref.** 8, pp. 1622, 1623)

653. E. The increased metabolic rate of children enhances the severity of carbon monoxide intoxication, leading to an earlier development of symptoms and possible death. (**Ref.** 1, p. 735; **Ref.** 6, pp. 1631–1633)

654. E. The administration of sympathomimetics in carbon tetrachloride poisoning is contraindicated because of hydrocarbon sensitization of the myocardium and the danger of producing severe arrhythmias. (**Ref.** 1, p. 737; **Ref.** 6, pp. 382, 1635)

655. E. The greater danger of lead poisoning in children than in adults is due primarily to the increased likelihood for the development of encephalopathy, but it may also be related to the far greater degree of absorption of lead when ingested by children. (**Ref.** 1, pp. 745–747; **Ref.** 3, pp. 729–730; **Ref.** 6, pp. 1606–1608, 1610)

656. B. The symptoms of chronic mercury poisoning vary with the type of mercury; the most consistent and pronounced effects of exposure to elemental mercury vapor and organic compounds are on the CNS, while the kidney is the primary target of inorganic mercury. (**Ref.** 1, pp. 748–749; **Ref.** 6, pp. 1611–1613; **Ref.** 8, p. 1600)

657. D. Although arsenic readily crosses the placental barrier, it passes the blood–brain barrier only with difficulty, brain levels of the metal being among the lowest in the body. (**Ref.** 1, pp. 747–748; **Ref.** 8, p. 1603)

658. D. These insecticides are potent anticholinesterase inhibitors which are diluted before use. Those who dilute these products may become acutely intoxicated from several drops of these insecticides on the skin. The toxic effects include bronchoconstriction. (**Ref.** 1, pp. 738–739; **Ref.** 8, p. 1629)

659. B. The PCBs and other chlorinated products, like the dioxins, can produce skin changes on contact including chloracne. (**Ref.** 1, p. 740)

660. C. Severe carbon monoxide poisoning requires immediate treatment to maintain respiration and oxygenation of the tissues after removal from the exposure site. (**Ref.** 1, p. 735; **Ref.** 8, p. 1620)

661. C. Effects of arsenic on the blood include leukopenia and eosinophilia, but not polycythemia. (**Ref.** 8, pp. 1603–1604)

662. C. Deferoxamine binds iron in preference to trace metals and does not remove iron from tissues but instead removes the loosely bound iron of the plasma. (**Ref.** 1, p. 744; **Ref.** 8, pp. 1291, 1611–1612)

663. A. This drug is used to remove arsenic and mercuric ions from the body and it has been used to remove lead from children. (**Ref.** 1, p. 744; **Ref.** 6, pp. 1621–1623; **Ref.** 8, pp. 1597–1598, 1604, 1609–1610)

11 Drug Interactions

DIRECTIONS (Questions 664–670): Each of the questions or incomplete statements below is followed by five suggested answers or completions. Select the **one** that is best in each case.

664. Clofibrate
   A. increases the likelihood of the formation of gallstones
   B. decreases and delays the absorption of chlorothiazide
   C. delays the absorption of tetracycline
   D. decreases the absorption of digitoxin
   E. when given to patients receiving dicumerol, the dose of dicumerol should be increased by 30% to 50%

665. Two drugs competing for plasma proteins thereby elevating the free (active) drug levels and causing enhanced, sometimes severe, effects are
   A. morphine and chlorpromazine
   B. aspirin and tolbutamine
   C. digoxin and hydrochlorothiazide
   D. diphenhydramine and reserpine
   E. probenecid and penicillin

666. Which one of the following drugs increases the metabolism of bishydroxycoumarin by induction of hepatic microsomal enzymes?
   A. Phenobarbital
   B. Methyldopa
   C. Phenylbutazone
   D. Thyroxine
   E. Guanethidine

667. All of the following adverse effects associated with the cited drug combinations have been observed EXCEPT
   A. respiratory paralysis: neomycin + ether
   B. cardiac arrhythmias: digitalis + reserpine
   C. hypertensive crisis: minoxidil + hydrochlorothiazide
   D. hypoglycemia reaction: tolbutamide + sulfisoxazole
   E. hemorrhagic episodes: warfarin + phenylbutazone

668. Inhibition of liver microsomal enzymes can lead to a long half-life for a drug. Which of the following have increased effectiveness when used with allopurinol, which inhibits liver microsomal enzymes?
   A. Aspirin
   B. Mercaptopurine
   C. Digoxin
   D. Ethanol
   E. Disulfiram

669. Absorption of oral drugs may be lowered or delayed by all of the following drug characteristics EXCEPT
   A. has a large surface area such as charcoal
   B. binds to drugs such as food and penicillin
   C. increases gastrointestinal emptying
   D. chelates to drugs such as milk
   E. none of the above

670. Combined toxicity may occur when two or more drugs have the same target organ or site of action. Which of the following combinations may lead to toxicity?

    A. Therapeutic dose of a benzodiazepine followed by several drinks of whiskey

    B. Loop acting diuretic combined with a thiazide diuretic

    C. Potassium and hydrochlorothiazide

    D. An aminoglycoside combined with a penicillin

    E. Therapeutic dose of probenicid followed by a therapeutic dose of benzylpenicillin

---

DIRECTIONS (Questions 671–689): Each group of questions below consists of five lettered headings followed by a list of numbered words, phrases, or statements. For each numbered word, phrase, or statement, select the **one** lettered heading that is most closely associated with it. Each lettered heading may be selected once, more than once, or not at all.

Questions 671–672:

    A. Sodium chloride
    B. Methenamine
    C. Chlorpromazine
    D. Clofibrate
    E. Tetracycline

671. Can block or reverse the pressor effect of epinephrine

672. Milk ingested within less than 2 hours of the time this drug is taken interferes with its absorption

Question 673:

    A. Verapamil
    B. Phenobarbital
    C. 6-Mercaptopurine
    D. Methotrexate
    E. Metronidazole

673. After drinking two alcoholic drinks (Manhattans) a severe pulsating headache and nausea are present, the pulse is rapid and weak, thirst and syncope occur (an antabuse-like reaction)

Questions 674-676:

A. Glucagon
B. Calcium
C. Furosemide
D. Pyridoxine
E. Disulfiram

674. Reduces levodopa-induced improvement in parkinsonism

675. Potentiates the hypokalemia from cortisol therapy

676. Patient taking metronidazole with this drug may develop changes including psychosis

Questions 677-680:

A. Cholestyramine
B. Hydrochlorothiazide
C. Propranolol
D. Quinidine
E. Large doses of aspirin

677. Can cause hyperuricemia and precipitate an acute attack of gout

678. Increases the effects of cardiac glycosides on cardiac excitability

679. Can potentiate digitalis-induced bradycardia

680. Reduces the absorption of orally administered digoxin

Questions 681–689:

    A. Patient taking propranolol
    B. Patient taking aspirin
    C. Patient digitalized with digitoxin
    D. Patient taking oral contraceptives
    E. Patient given meperidine

681. Heparin should never be given to patient taking this drug

682. Taking hydroxyzine may cause serious respiratory depression by this drug

683. When patient takes griseofulvin may no longer be effective

684. Thiazide diuretics added to the therapy will increase the effect of this drug and may lead to toxic effects

685. Reserpine given parenterally may cause arrhythmias in patient taking this drug

686. An alteration in the bacterial flora of the intestines will reduce the effectiveness of this drug

687. Taking cimetidine with this drug may lead to bradycardia

688. Acidifying the urine with ammonium chloride given orally may slow the excretion of this drug, prolonging its action

689. Taking quinidine makes this drug more effective and may lead to toxic effects

---

DIRECTIONS (Questions 690–693): The set of lettered headings below is followed by a list of numbered words or phrases. For each numbered word or phrase select

    A if the item is associated with **A** only
    B if the item is associated with **B** only
    C if the item is associated with both **A** and **B**
    D if the item is associated with neither **A** nor **B**

    A. Therapeutic effects are reduced
    B. Therapeutic effects are increased or even toxic effects may occur
    C. Both
    D. Neither

690. Five days after discontinuing tranylcypromine, the patient started taking impramine

691. Individual taking tranylcypromine ate a cheeseburger and drank some beer

692. Change in phenytoin effects when phenobarbital is added to the therapy

693. Monoamine oxidase inhibitor is given to patient taking an oral antidiabetic drug

---

DIRECTIONS (Questions 694–700): For each of the questions or incomplete statements below, **one** or **more** of the answers or completions given is correct. Select

    A if only 1, 2, and 3 are correct
    B if only 1 and 3 are correct
    C if only 2 and 4 are correct
    D if only 4 is correct
    E if all are correct

---

694. Adverse drug interactions may occur due to alteration in
    1. absorption
    2. excretion
    3. distribution
    4. pharmacodynamics

695. Mechanisms responsible for drug interactions include
   1. enzyme induction
   2. increase of chemical transmitter at receptors
   3. depletion or reduction of transmitter at receptors
   4. inhibition of protein synthesis

696. The sites for plasma protein binding include
   1. albumin
   2. transferrin
   3. globulin
   4. α and β lipoproteins

697. Drug half-life can be prolonged by
   1. decreased activity of enzymes responsible for its metabolism
   2. increased amount deposited in adipose tissue
   3. reduced liver and kidney function
   4. decreased amount bound to plasma proteins

698. Epinephrine and theophylline contribute to increased cyclic AMP by the influence of
   1. epinephrine on phosphodiesterase
   2. epinephrine on adenyl cyclase
   3. theophylline on adenyl cyclase
   4. theophylline on phosphodiesterase

699. Digoxin absorption is altered by
   1. use of an antibiotic
   2. use of a potassium-depleting drug
   3. use of penicillamine
   4. use of a bile acid-binding resin

700. Carbamazepine will induce the drug-metabolizing enzymes of the liver thereby increasing the metabolism of
   1. ampicillin
   2. haloperidol
   3. atenolol
   4. corticosteroids

Explanatory Answers

664. A. Clofibrate increases hepatic excretion of cholesterol, and therefore may elevate cholesterol concentration in bile, and increases twofold to threefold the possibility of gallstone formation. (**Ref.** 1, p. 426; **Ref.** 2, p. 341; **Ref.** 8, p. 889; **Ref.** 9, p. 246)

665. B. Of those listed, only aspirin and tolbutamide produce enhanced effects by competition for plasma protein binding, which results in higher free (active) drug levels and hypoglycemia. (**Ref.** 1, p. 838; **Ref.** 3, p. 741; **Ref.** 6, p. 679; **Ref.** 8, pp. 1485–1487; **Ref.** 9, p. 949)

666. A. Of the drugs listed, only phenobarbital causes induction of hepatic enzymes, which is involved in the metabolism of coumarins, thereby reducing the effects of the anticoagulants unless the dose is increased. Other drugs with similar action are meprobamate, chloral hydrate, glutethimide, and griseofulvin. (**Ref.** 1, pp. 411, 834; **Ref.** 3, p. 741; **Ref.** 6, p. 1356; **Ref.** 8, p. 362; **Ref.** 9, p. 949)

667. C. Minoxidil is useful in the treatment of hypertension crises as it causes dilation of arterioles by its direct action. It is necessary to give a diuretic with it because minoxidil causes sodium retention. The other listed adverse effects can occur with drugs as stated. (**Ref.** 3, p. 196; **Ref.** 6, pp. 1347–1348; **Ref.** 8, pp. 802–803; **Ref.** 9, p. 278)

668. BC. Mercaptopurine has a small margin of safety and when used with allopurinol the dose must be reduced because allopurinol interferes with the metabolism of mercaptopurine. (**Ref.** 1, p. 832; **Ref.** 8, p. 677; **Ref.** 9, p. 599)

669. E. Charcoal is used as an antidote for overdose of oral drugs. Certain components of food can bind strongly to drugs, especially the weak acids such as benylpenicillin. Oral drugs are less effective when the intestinal contents turn over more rapidly. (**Ref.** 1, p. 831; **Ref.** 8, p. 57; **Ref.** 9, p. 29)

670. A. Alcohol and benzodiazepines have formed many a lethal mixture for the unwary due to the combined depressant effects. (**Ref.** 1, pp. 101, 189, 832, 837; **Ref.** 8, p. 376; **Ref.** 9, p. 540)

671. C. Chlorpromazine, in addition to many other pharmacologic-blocking properties, possesses appreciable α-adrenergic blocking actions and can consequently block or reverse the pressor effects of epinephrine. (**Ref.** 6, p. 399)

672. E. Milk contains calcium salts, which chelate with tetracycline if each are taken together or about the same time. Chelated tetracycline is not absorbed. (**Ref.** 1, p. 568; **Ref.** 2, p. 694; **Ref.** 3, pp. 645, 737; **Ref.** 6, p. 1054; **Ref.** 8, p. 1004; **Ref.** 9, p. 540)

673. E. Metronidazole interferes with completion of the metabolism of alcohol, allowing acetaldehyde to accumulate; this causes antabuse-like symptoms, many of which are related to the pronounced vasodilation. (**Ref.** 1, p. 662; **Ref.** 2, p. 732; **Ref.** 8, p. 1004; **Ref.** 9, p. 540)

674. D. Acting as a coenzyme, pyridoxine increases the decarboxylase activity in the body, accelerates the conversion of L-dopa to dopamine in the periphery, and thus makes less L-dopa available for penetration into the CNS. (**Ref.** 1, p. 836; **Ref.** 2, p. 575; **Ref.** 3, p. 137; **Ref.** 6, pp. 479–480)

675. C. Although furosemide increases and corticosterone decreases sodium excretion, both drugs cause a urinary loss of body potassium. (**Ref.** 1, pp. 188–189; **Ref.** 3, pp. 488, 531; **Ref.** 6, pp. 867, 871–872, 897; **Ref.** 8, pp. 723–724; **Ref.** 9, pp. 269–270)

676. E. By an unknown mechanism metronidazole and disulfiram used together have produced psychoses. Both of these drugs will interact with a number of other drugs, usually by known mechanisms. (**Ref.** 1, p. 836)

677. B. Hydrochlorothiazide in some patients reduces uric acid excretion sufficiently to precipitate an attack of gout. Aspirin in large doses has an uricosuric action. (**Ref.** 1, p. 190; **Ref.** 3, pp. 574–575; **Ref.** 6, pp. 713, 895; **Ref.** 8, p. 647)

678. B. Thiazides can cause hypokalemia, which increases the actions of cardiac glycosides. Furosemide, corticosteroids, and large infusions of glucose have this same effect. (**Ref.** 1, pp. 189–190; **Ref.** 2, p. 354; **Ref.** 3, p. 486; **Ref.** 6, p. 738; **Ref.** 8, p. 721; **Ref.** 9, p. 265)

679. C. Propranolol's β-adrenergic blocking action on the heart produces a pronounced bradycardia. (**Ref.** 1, p. 129; **Ref.** 2, pp. 189–190; **Ref.** 3, pp. 207, 405; **Ref.** 6, pp. 198, 743)

680. A. Cholestyramine, an anion-exchange resin, binds digoxin in the intestine to reduce its availability. (**Ref.** 1, p. 834; **Ref.** 2, pp. 336–337; **Ref.** 6, pp. 733, 841; **Ref.** 8, p. 891; **Ref.** 9, p. 241)

681. B. Aspirin inhibits aggregation of platelets and this would markedly prolong bleeding time in the presence of heparin. (**Ref.** 1, p. 434; **Ref.** 2, pp. 428–429; **Ref.** 6, p. 683; **Ref.** 8, p. 1325; **Ref.** 9, p. 379)

682. E. Hydroxyzine potentiates many of the actions of the opiates and opioids including analgesic, hypnotic, and respiratory depressant actions. (**Ref.** 2, p. 531; **Ref.** 6, p. 508)

683. D. Griseofulvin inhibits the effectiveness of the oral contraceptives by an unknown mechanism. (**Ref.** 1, p. 836; **Ref.** 8, p. 1174; **Ref.** 9, p. 890)

684. C. A fall in the serum potassium greatly increases the effectiveness of the cardiac glycosides and can add to the toxicity. (**Ref.** 1, pp. 835–836; **Ref.** 9, p. 315)

685. C. Reserpine releases catecholamines, which may cause arrhythmias in a digitalized patient. (**Ref.** 3, p. 429)

686. D. Estrogens in the oral contraceptives are continuously removed by the liver and then reabsorbed from the intestines. This enterohepatic circulation of the estrogens is altered by diarrhea, especially when the intestinal bacterial flora is changed. (**Ref.** 1, p. 836; **Ref.** 9, pp. 874, 890)

687. A. Propranolol metabolism is slowed when the liver microsomal enzymes are inhibited by cimetidine. (**Ref.** 1, p. 834)

688. B. Aspirin is excreted more slowly and its action would be prolonged since only 2% is excreted in acid urine as salicylates while over 30% is excreted in alkaline urine. (**Ref.** 8, p. 650)

689. C. Digitalized patients must have their dose adjusted when quinidine is added to their therapy. Quinidine both displaces digoxin from the plasma protein and reduces the renal loss of digoxin. (**Ref.** 1, p. 836; **Ref.** 3, p. 429; **Ref.** 8, p. 836; **Ref.** 9, p. 317)

690. B. Toxic effects can be expected from intense adrenergic activity because tricyclic antidepressant blocks norepinephrine uptake and 10 to 14 days are required for the synthesis of new MAO after discontinuation of MAO inhibitors. (**Ref.** 2, pp. 530–531; **Ref.** 6, pp. 422, 426; **Ref.** 8, p. 417; **Ref.** 9, p. 484)

691. B. Tyramine is present in such foods as cheese, beer, liver, and sour cream. Many over-the-counter cold, hay fever, and weight-reducing products contain adrenergic amines. Toxic effects include tachycardia, hypertension, hypotension and collapse, hyperpyrexia, and convulsions. (**Ref.** 2, p. 554)

692. C. Phenobarbital can induce microsomal enzymes as well as compete with phenytoin for these enzymes. Therefore, phenytoin effects can be increased, decreased, or unchanged. (**Ref.** 2, pp. 564–565; **Ref.** 6, p. 358; **Ref.** 8, p. 445; **Ref.** 9, p. 493)

693. B. Currently available MAO inhibitors have an intrinsic hypoglycemic effect which is additive to the oral antidiabetic drugs. (**Ref.** 1, p. 837)

694. E. Adverse drug reactions may result from competition for and/or modification of many mechanisms such as absorption, distribution, protein binding, receptor availability, and enzyme transformation. (**Ref.** 1, p. 831; **Ref.** 3, p. 737; **Ref.** 6, pp. 54–55; **Ref.** 9, p. 318)

695. E. Additional factors contributing to drug interactions include modified uptake of drug at the receptor site, modified absorption, modified excretion, modified electrolytes, and inhibition of the metabolic process. (**Ref.** 1, p. 831; **Ref.** 3, pp. 737–739; **Ref.** 6, pp. 1734–1736)

696. E. Drugs may be bound to one or more of these substances in plasma. After binding sites become saturated, the amount of free drug increases by a quantity, depending on the amounts administered. (**Ref.** 2, pp. 34–35; **Ref.** 3, p. 22; **Ref.** 6, pp. 12, 1735)

697. A. The drug bound to plasma proteins and that deposited in adipose tissue constitute a reservoir from which the drug is slowly released. As the plasma-free drug concentration tends to fall, the drug is released from these reservoirs, causing prolonged half-life. (**Ref.** 2, pp. 34–35; **Ref.** 3, p. 21; **Ref.** 6, pp. 27–28)

698. C. Adenyl cyclase increases the conversion of ATP to cyclic AMP; β-adrenergic agonists activate this enzyme. Phosphodiesterase inhibition by theophylline reduces or prevents the loss of cyclic AMP into 5′-AMP. (**Ref.** 3, pp. 161–162; **Ref.** 6, pp. 88–89)

699. D. Digoxin absorption is altered by the bile acid-binding resins. These resins are eliminated essentially unchanged and will take the digoxin with them. (**Ref.** 1, p. 836; **Ref.** 9, pp. 318, 379)

700. C. Both haloperidol and corticosteroids are metabolized by the drug-metabolizing enzymes of the liver. Ampicillin and atenolol are excreted to a very large extent by the kidneys (82% and 94%, respectively). (**Ref.** 1, p. 385; **Ref.** 8, pp. 237, 1069, 1658, 1659; **Ref.** 9, p. 469)

References

1. Katzung BG: *Basic and Clinical Pharmacology*, 4th Ed. Norwalk, CT, San Mateo, CA, Appleton and Lange, 1989.

2. Craig CR, Stitzel RE: *Modern Pharmacology*, 2nd Ed. Boston, Little, Brown, 1986.

3. Clark WG, Brater DC, Johnson AR: *Goth's Medical Pharmacology*, 12th Ed. St. Louis, CV Mosby, 1988.

4. Barkow R (Ed): *The Merck Manual*, 15th Ed. West Point, PA, Merck, Sharp and Dohme, 1987.

5. *Physicians' Desk Reference*, 44th Ed. Oradell, NJ, Medical Economic Co., 1990.

6. Gilman AG, Goodman LS, Rall TW, Murad F: *The Pharmacological Basis of Therapeutics*, 7th Ed. New York, Macmillan, 1985.

7. *Drug Evaluation*, 6th Ed. Chicago, American Medical Association, 1986.

8. Gilman AG, Rall TW, Nies AS, Taylor P: *The Pharmacological Basis of Therapeutics*, 8th Ed. New York, Pergamon Press, 1990.

9. Craig CR, Stitzel RE: *Modern Pharmacology*, 3rd Ed. Boston, Little, Brown, 1990.

10. Furman PA, et al: Phosphorylation of 3-azido-3-deoxythymidine and selective interaction of the 5-tri-phosphate with human immunodeficiency virus reverse transcriptase. *Proc Natl Acad Sci USA* 1986;83:8333–8337.

11. McKinley MA, Rossman MG: Rational design of antiviral agents. *Annu Rev Pharmacol* 1989;29:111.

12. Antimicrobial prophylaxis in surgery, *Medical Letter*, December 1, 1989; 31:105–108.

13. Sarin PS: Molecular pharmacologic approaches to the treatment of AIDS. *Annu Rev Pharmacol* 1988;28:411–428.

14. Mannerung GJ, Deloris LB: Pharmacology and toxicology of the interferons. *Annu Rev Pharmacol* 1986;26:455–515.

15. Fischl MA: The efficacy of azidothymidine in the treatment of patients with AIDS and AIDS-related complex. *N Engl J Med* 1987;316:185–191.

16. Rakel RE (Ed): *Conn's Current Therapy*. Philadelphia, WB Saunders, 1990.

17. Lehninger AL: *Biochemistry*, 2nd Ed. New York, Worth Publishers, 1975.

18. Rakel RE (Ed): *Conn's Current Therapy*. Philadelphia, WB Saunders, 1989.